Diagnosis and Management of Type 2 Diabetes

Fifth Edition

Steven V. Edelman, MD

Professor of Medicine
Division of Endocrinology and Metabolism
University of California, San Diego

Robert R. Henry, MD

Professor of Medicine
Division of Endocrinology and Metabolism
University of California, San Diego

SO-AHF-591

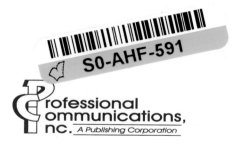

Professional
Communications,
Inc. _A Publishing Corporation_

Published by
Professional Communications, Inc.

Marketing Office:
400 Center Bay Drive
West Islip, NY 11795
(t) 631/661-2852
(f) 631/661-2167

Editorial Office:
PO Box 10
Caddo, OK   74729-0010
(t) 580/367-9838
(f) 580/367-9989

ISBN: 1-884735-75-4
Printed in the United States of America

For orders only, please call:
1-800-337-9838
Or visit our website:
www.pcibooks.com

DISCLAIMER
The opinions expressed in this publication reflect those of the authors. However, the authors make no warranty regarding the contents of the publication. The protocols described herein are general and may not apply to a specific patient. Any product mentioned in this publication should be taken in accordance with the prescribing information provided by the manufacturer.

This text is printed on recycled paper.

ii

DEDICATION

To our wives, Ingrid and Denine,
and our children, Talia, Carina,
Ryan, Danny, and Dustin,
for their tolerance and patience during
the writing of this book.

ACKNOWLEDGMENT

The authors thank the many individuals who have been a major force shaping the field of diabetes and influencing their opinions.

We would like also to express our appreciation to Phyllis Freeny for her excellent editorial assistance and Nikki D. Weaver for her exceptional graphics design work. Our assistants, George Rivera and Sue Pryor, are invaluable sources of help. Lastly, we would like to thank Malcolm Beasley for his patience and unyielding support in writing this book.

TABLE OF CONTENTS

Part 1 *General Information*	**Diabetes Statistics**	1
	Pathophysiology and Natural History	2
Part 2 *Diagnosis*	**Classification**	3
	Diagnosis of Diabetes and the Metabolic Syndrome	4
Part 3 *Nonpharmacologic Treatment*	**Nutrition**	5
	Exercise	6
Part 4 *Pharmacologic Treatment*	**Oral Agents**	7
	Insulin Therapy	8
Part 5 *Treatment Assessment*	**Treatment Algorithm**	9
	Assessment of the Treatment Regimen	10
Part 6 *Complications*	**Acute Complications**	11
	Long-term Complications	12
Part 7 *Resources*	**Resources**	13
Index		14

TABLES

Table 3.1   Distinguishing Characteristics of
Diabetes Mellitus and Other Disorders
of Glucose Intolerance 30

Table 3.2   Diagnostic Criteria for Impaired Fasting
Glucose and Impaired Glucose Tolerance
Using the Oral Glucose Tolerance Test 34

Table 4.1   Normal Plasma Glucose Values for
Nonpregnant Adults 40

Table 4.2   Criteria for the Diagnosis of
Diabetes Mellitus...41

Table 4.3   Clinical Criteria of the
Metabolic Syndrome 48

Table 4.4   Major and Minor Criteria for the
Dysmetabolic Syndrome X 49

Table 5.1   Suggested Weight for Adults 55

Table 5.2   Practical Dietary Recommendations 58

Table 6.1   General Exercise Guidelines 67

Table 6.2   Practical Exercise Prescription 68

Table 7.1   Suggested Glycemic Guidelines 73

Table 7.2   United Kingdom Prospective Diabetes Study:
Intensive Blood-Glucose Control 74

Table 7.3   Characteristics of Currently Available
Oral Antidiabetic Agents 82

Table 7.4   Acarbose/Miglitol Dosing Instructions
for Patients 100

Table 8.1   Time Course of Action of
Insulin Preparations 126

Table 8.2   Common Insulin Regimens
Used in Adult Diabetes 128

Table 8.3   Guidelines for Dosing Insulin in
Combination Therapy 132

Table 8.4   Patient Self Adjustment of
Evening Insulin 133

Table 8.5   Stepwise Approach for Initiating a
Split-Mixed Insulin Regimen in Patients
With Type 2 Diabetes................................... 137

Table 9.1   Glycemic Control for People
                   With Diabetes 150

Table 10.1   Metabolic Goals of
                   Effective Management 156

Table 10.2   Blood Glucose Meters: Specifications 166

Table 10.3   Blood Glucose Meters: Features 170

Table 10.4   Techniques Used to Adjust for
                   Premeal Hyperglycemia 177

Table 10.5   Patient Self Adjustment of Insulin
                   Dosage, Split-Mixed Regimen 184

Table 11.1   Symptoms and Signs of Classic
                   Diabetic Ketoacidosis 192

Table 11.2   Initial Laboratory Values for Patients
                   Experiencing Diabetic Ketoacidosis 194

Table 11.3   Diabetic Ketoacidosis and Hyperglycemic
                   Hyperosmolar Nonketotic Syndrome:
                   Comparison of Some Salient Features 200

Table 11.4   Infections Common or Special to Patients
                   With Diabetes Mellitus 208

Table 12.1   Potential Complications of Common
                   Antihypertensive Agents
                   in the Patient With Diabetes 215

Table 12.2   Potential Benefits of Common
                   Antihypertensive Agents 216

Table 12.3   Lipid Levels for Adults 221

Table 12.4   Treatment Decisions Based
                   on LDL Cholesterol Level in
                   Adults With Diabetes 222

Table 12.5   Diet Recommendations for the Treatment
                   of Lipid Disorders in Diabetes 224

Table 12.6   Order of Priorities for Treatment of
                   Diabetic Dyslipidemia in Adults 225

Table 12.7   Pharmacologic Agents for Treatment
                   of Dyslipidemia in Adults 226

Table 12.8   Reasons to Refer Patients With Type 2
                   Diabetes Mellitus to an Eye Doctor 233

Table 12.9   Types of Diabetic Neuropathies 238

Table 12.10   Care of the Diabetic Foot 250

vii

FIGURES

Figure 1.1   Percentage of the Population With
              Diagnosed Diabetes, By Age and Sex,
              United States, 1995-1997 12

Figure 1.2   Incidence of Diabetes per 1000 Population,
              By Age and Sex, 1995-1997 13

Figure 1.3   Percentage Prevalence of Diabetes
              By State, 1996 14

Figure 1.4   Percentage of the US Population ≥20
              Years of Age With Diagnosed Diabetes,
              Undiagnosed Diabetes, and Impaired
              Fasting Glucose 15

Figure 1.5   Approximate Distribution of Causes of
              Death in People With Diabetes, Based
              on US Studies 17

Figure 2.1   The Natural History of Type 2 Diabetes 23

Figure 4.1   Diabetes Warranty Program 44

Figure 7.1   United Kingdom Prospective Diabetes
              Study Cross-Sectional and 10-Year
              Cohort Data for HbA_{1C}: Intensive or
              Conventional Treatment 75

Figure 7.2   Change in Fasting Plasma Glucose
              Concentrations at Week 26 in
              Patients Taking Metformin and
              Rosiglitazone Compared With Taking
              Metformin Alone 87

Figure 7.3   Mean Fasting Plasma Glucose
              Concentrations Over Time in Patients
              Taking Metformin Alone Compared
              With Patients Taking Metformin
              and Rosiglitazone 88

Figure 7.4   Dose-Dependent Reduction in Fasting
              Plasma Glucose Concentrations With
              Pioglitazone Added to Insulin 92

Figure 7.5   Comparison of Nateglinide on PPG
              Levels Following Sustacal Challenge 109

Figure 8.1   Fast-Acting Insulin Analogs: Lispro
              (Humalog) and Aspart (Novolog) 123

Figure 8.2   Peak Action of Insulin Compared With
                Peak Rise in Glucose After Eating 127

Figure 9.1   Treatment Algorithm for Pharmacologic
                Therapy of Type 2 Diabetes 152

Figure 10.1   Cooperative Relationship Between
                Fructosamine and HbA_{1C} Values 161

Figure 10.2   Weekly Self-Monitoring Blood
                Glucose Record Sheet 180

Figure 10.3   Algorithm Form Used for Patients
                on Intensive Insulin Therapy 182

Figure 12.1   Background Diabetic Retinopathy 230

Figure 12.2   Preproliferative Retinopathy 231

Figure 12.3   Managing Painful Diabetic Neuropathy ... 241

1 Diabetes Statistics

The prevalence and incidence of type 2 diabetes is increasing not only in the United States, but also around the world. The prevalence of diabetes refers to the total number of people known to have the disease at a particular time. In 1997, 16 million Americans (6% of the US population) had diabetes. Approximately one third of those individuals were estimated to have undiagnosed diabetes. The prevalence has increased from 4.9% in 1990 to approximately 6.5% documented in 1998. Possible reasons for the substantial increases in the prevalence of diabetes over time include:

- Advancing age of the US population
- Reduced diabetic mortality rates due to improved screening, detection, and healthcare
- An increase in risk factors such as obesity and physical inactivity.

The prevalence of diabetes increases with advancing age reaching nearly 12% for those in the age 65 to 74 category (Figure 1.1). The prevalence is similar for men and women up to age of 65 and for those over 65, the prevalence rates are slightly higher for men. Although the prevalence rates of diagnosed diabetes are equal for men and women, 45% of all people with diabetes are male and 55% are female (Figure 1.2). The prevalence of individuals with type 2 diabetes is considerably different depending on the race and ethnicity in the US population (Figure 1.3). Diabetes is more prevalent in African Americans, Latinos, Native American Indians, Pacific Islanders, and Indian Asians. The increasing number of ethnic minorities

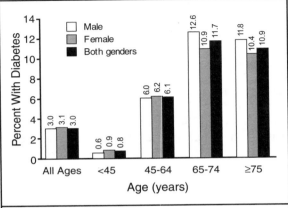

FIGURE 1.1 — PERCENTAGE OF THE POPULATION WITH DIAGNOSED DIABETES, BY AGE AND SEX, UNITED STATES, 1995-1997

Data are the average for 3 years 1995-1997; rates for both genders are age-adjusted to the 1980 US population.

American Diabetes Association: Diabetes statistics. *Diabetes 2001 Vital Statistics*; 2001:14.

in the United States may also contribute to the increasing prevalence of type 2 diabetes.

The lowering of the clinical diagnostic criteria for the diagnoses of diabetes from a fasting blood sugar of 140 mg/dL to 126 mg/dL has also contributed to the higher prevalence of diabetes. The ethnic minorities not only have a higher prevalence of diabetes, but they also have a greater number of individuals with undiagnosed diabetes as well as impaired fasting glucose, which is a risk factor for the development of type 2 diabetes. It has been estimated that 37% of all diabetics in the United States currently do not know they have the disease. The prevalence of undiagnosed diabetes also increases with age in both men and women. In the age 60 to 74 category, the rate of undiagnosed diabetes is estimated to be 6.2% (Figure 1.4).

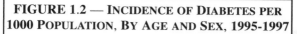

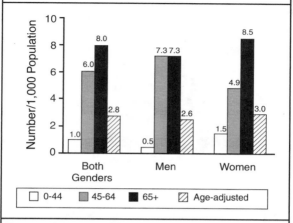

Data are the average for 3 years 1995-1997; rates for both genders are age-adjusted to the 1980 US population.

American Diabetes Association: Diabetes statistics. *Diabetes 2001 Vital Statistics*; 2001:18.

Undiagnosed type 2 diabetes is a serious problem. Insulin resistance and the associated macrovascular complications are well known to develop 10 to 15 years before the typical diagnosis of type 2 diabetes. In the United Kingdom Prospective Diabetes Study, 21% of the newly diagnosed diabetics had diabetic retinopathy. Since diabetic retinopathy requires at least 4 to 7 years of hyperglycemia to develop, this indicates that diabetes went undiagnosed for this period of time. In addition, these newly diagnosed subjects also had a two to three times higher incidence of myocardial infarction and stroke compared with the general population.

The incidence of diabetes is the number of new cases diagnosed during some period of time, usually in the previous year. According to the most recent es-

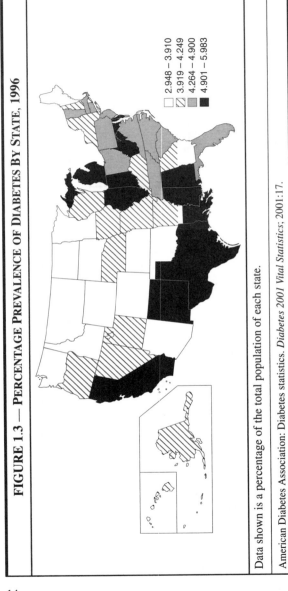

FIGURE 1.3 — PERCENTAGE PREVALENCE OF DIABETES BY STATE, 1996

☐	2.948 – 3.910
▨	3.919 – 4.249
▦	4.264 – 4.900
■	4.901 – 5.983

Data shown is a percentage of the total population of each state.

American Diabetes Association: Diabetes statistics. *Diabetes 2001 Vital Statistics*; 2001:17.

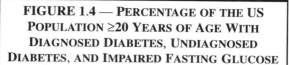

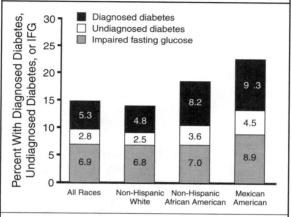

American Diabetes Association: Diabetes statistics. *Diabetes 2001 Vital Statistics*; 2001:17.

timate, approximately 780,000 individuals in the United States are diagnosed with diabetes each year (over 2,000 people per day). Approximately 42% of these people are between the ages of 45 and 64, with a greater percentage of new cases among women (57%) compared with men (43%). The average annual incidence rate for diagnosed diabetes is approximately 2.8 per 1,000 people with a slightly higher incidence for women.

The incidence rates for diagnosed diabetes increased by about 18% from 1980 to the current estimates. In a similar fashion to the prevalence, the incidence rates for African American, Latinos, Native American Indian, Pacific Islanders and Asian Indians are higher than for whites. Some experts believe that the increasing incidence of diabetes is due to a genetic predisposition to diabetes commonly referred to as

"The Thrifty Gene Hypothesis." The thrifty gene hypothesis theorizes that in the past, most individuals were hunters and gatherers doing physical labor for their daily existence. In times of famine, any individual that was not thin and had insulin resistance would be in a prime position to survive and not perish from starvation. In a relatively short period of time, individuals in our westernized societies are doing less physical labor, growing older, becoming much more obese, and consuming foods in greater amounts and with a much higher percentage of fat. What was a physiologic advantage in the past is now a physiologic disadvantage. All of these factors are thought to contribute to the increasing incidence of type 2 diabetes.

In conclusion, diabetes has achieved or is nearing epidemic proportion in many ethnic groups, not only in the United States, but also in other populations around the globe. Much of the increase is due to our westernized society lifestyle that contributes significantly to the overall morbidity and mortality associated with type 2 diabetes (Figure 1.5). In order to reduce the emotional and physical suffering of people with type 2 diabetes, a concerted effort should be undertaken towards the prevention, early detection, and aggressive management of this devastating condition.

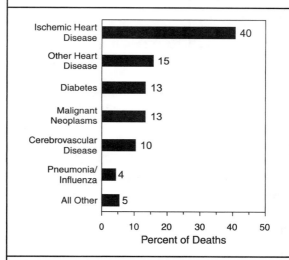

FIGURE 1.5 — APPROXIMATE DISTRIBUTION OF CAUSES OF DEATH IN PEOPLE WITH DIABETES, BASED ON US STUDIES

Geiss LS, Herman WH, Smith PJ. Mortality in non–insulin-dependent diabetes. In: Harris MI, Cowie CC, Stern MP, et al, eds. *Diabetes in America*. Bethesda, Md: National Institutes of Health, National Institutes of Diabetes and Digestive and Kidney Diseases; 1995:236-237.

SUGGESTED READING

Fagot-Gampagna A, Pettit DJ, Engelgau MM, et al. Type 2 diabetes among North American children and adolescents: an epidemiologic review and a public health perspective. *J Pediatr.* 2000;136:664-672.

Ramachandran A, Snehalatha C, Latha E, Vijay V, Viswanathan M. Rising prevalence of NIDDM in an urban population in India. *Diabetologia.* 1997;40:232-237.

Tan CE, Emmanuel SC, Tan BY, Jacob E. Prevalence of diabetes and ethnic differences in cardiovascular risk factors. The 1992 Singapore National Health Survey. *Diabetes Care.* 1999;22:241-247.

World Health Organization. Definition, diagnosis and classification of diabetes mellitus and its complications. Part 1: Diagnosis and classification of diabetes mellitus (Department of Noncommunicable Disease Surveillance, Geneva, 1999).

Zimmet P, Alberti KG, Shaw J. Global and societal implications of the diabetes epidemic. *Nature* 2001;414:782-787.

2

Pathophysiology and Natural History

Pathophysiology

Type 2 diabetes is known to have a strong genetic component with contributing environmental determinants. The genetic influence is readily apparent from data of twin and family studies. Identification of type 2 diabetes susceptibility genes has been elusive, and investigations of a number of candidate genes has been largely negative, yielding a very small population of patients (less than 5%) with genetic variation in any of the candidate genes studied to date.

It is likely that no single genetic defect will emerge to explain type 2 diabetes; thus, the disease is heterogeneous and probably multigenic, and likely has a complex etiology. Even though the disease is genetically heterogeneous, there appears to be a fairly consistent phenotype once the disease is fully manifested. Most patients with type 2 diabetes and fasting hyperglycemia are characterized by:

- Insulin resistance
- Impaired insulin secretion
- Increased hepatic glucose production.

Although these three metabolic abnormalities have been well studied and characterized, the etiologic sequence has only recently come into focus.

It is probable that the increased hepatic glucose production of type 2 diabetes is secondary and can be fully reversed with a variety of forms of antidiabetic therapy. In addition, increased hepatic glucose production rates do not exist in the state of impaired glucose tolerance

(IGT). This leaves insulin resistance, impaired insulin secretion, or both, as initiating abnormalities.

Recent accumulated evidence strongly supports the idea that both insulin resistance and impaired insulin secretion precede the onset of hyperglycemia and the type 2 diabetes phenotype. However, insulin resistance is quantitatively more severe in the prediabetic phenotype. In fact, studies have also shown that insulin secretion, including first-phase insulin responses to intravenous glucose, are either normal or increased in the prediabetic or IGT state. Thus, substantial evidence from the literature indicates that those individuals who evolve from IGT to type 2 diabetes begin with insulin resistance.

Although genetic factors underlie the etiology of type 2 diabetes in most patients, acquired factors may also be contributory, such as:

- Obesity, particularly central or visceral obesity
- Sedentary lifestyle
- High-fat diets.

The aging process also contributes to the expression of type 2 diabetes in genetically susceptible individuals. When the β-cell function is able to compensate for insulin resistance, hyperinsulinemia develops, which maintains relatively normal glucose tolerance. Therefore, in the compensated insulin-resistant, hyperinsulinemic state, one has either normal glucose tolerance or IGT, but not diabetes. A subpopulation of individuals with compensated insulin resistance eventually go on to develop type 2 diabetes. The magnitude of this subpopulation depends on the methods used to detect glucose intolerance, the particular ethnic groups studied, and several other acquired and metabolic abnormalities that may be present. In addition, during the transition from the compensated state to frank type 2 diabetes, at least three pathophysiologic changes can be observed:

20

- First, basal hepatic glucose production rates increase, which is a characteristic feature of essentially all type 2 diabetes patients with fasting hyperglycemia.
- Second, the insulin resistance usually becomes more severe, which may be due to the degree of genetic load and/or acquired conditions such as obesity, sedentary lifestyle, and aging. Antidiabetic treatment can completely normalize the elevated hepatic glucose production rates and partially ameliorate the insulin resistance so that the degree of insulin resistance returns approximately to the level present in the IGT state. Thus, increased hepatic output and the worsening of insulin resistance are likely to be secondary phenomena.
- The third and most marked change is a decrease in β-cell function and decline in insulin secretory ability. Whether this decline in insulin secretion is because of preprogrammed genetic abnormalities in β-cell function or acquired defects such as glucose toxicity or β-cell exhaustion, or both, remains to be elucidated. Nevertheless, a marked decrease in β-cell function accompanies this transition and is thought to be a major contributor to the transition from IGT to type 2 diabetes.

In summary, the proposed etiologic sequence is that insulin resistance (probably genetic in origin) and abnormalities of pancreatic insulin secretion are manifested initially. The pancreas tries to compensate for insulin resistance which leads to increased insulin secretion to maintain the prediabetic state. In time, the compensation fails and β-cell function declines, leading to hyperglycemia. Note, however, that most type 2 diabetic patients, particularly the majority which are obese at the time of initial diagnosis, are still hyperinsulinemic. In addition, the conversion of IGT to type 2 diabetes can also be influenced by:

- Ethnicity
- Degree of obesity
- Distribution of body fat
- Sedentary lifestyle
- Aging
- Other concomitant medical conditions.

The heterogeneous nature of type 2 diabetes and its natural history result in the varied response to the different antidiabetic agents over time.

The Natural History of Diabetes

Type 2 diabetes is at one end of the continuum represented by the fully compensated insulin-resistant state to IGT to frank type 2 diabetes. A triad of metabolic defects characterizes type 2 diabetes: insulin resistance, non-autoimmune β-cell dysfunction, and inappropriately increased hepatic glucose production (Figure 2.1). The natural history of type 2 diabetes directly reflects the interrelationships between these three defects. The primary and earliest pathogenic lesion is insulin resistance and the β-cell is able to compensate for a variable length of time by secreting supraphysiologic amounts of insulin. Insulin resistance, compensatory hyperinsulinemia, and mild postprandial hyperglycemia characterize IGT. Over time, however, the β-cell begins to fail and as relative insulin deficiency occurs, fasting hyperglycemia and full-blown type 2 diabetes develops. In addition, as insulin levels fall, the inhibitory effect of insulin on hepatic glucose production decreases and significant fasting hyperglycemia develops. Further progression of the disease is marked by an absolute insulin deficiency. Obesity, aging, weight gain in adulthood, and physical inactivity are some of the environmental fac-

FIGURE 2.1 — THE NATURAL HISTORY OF TYPE 2 DIABETES

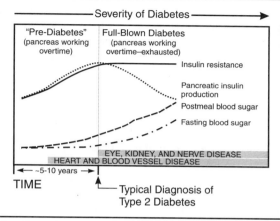

Insulin resistance can be present for many years before the diagnosis of diabetes. Blood sugar levels are not markedly elevated in the early stages of diabetes. Once the pancreas becomes exhausted, blood sugar values increase dramatically. As the pancreas becomes exhausted, the chance of achieving good glucose control with diet and exercise alone or with one oral agent is reduced.

Source: Edelman SV. *Taking Control of Your Diabetes*. 2nd ed. Caddo, Okla: Professional Communications, Inc; 2001.

tors that impact the natural history of diabetes, affecting its progression at all points in the continuum.

Screening patients for IGT is probably the best way for early identification of high-risk individuals since postprandial hyperglycemia occurs typically before the onset of fasting hyperglycemia in the natural history of type 2 diabetes. However, the diagnosis of IGT requires that an oral glucose tolerance test be performed. This procedure is cumbersome and has largely been replaced by fasting plasma glucose testing in general clinical practice because of convenience and greater reproducibility. This change in practice patterns underscores the importance of the new impaired fasting glucose (IFG) criteria (ie, glucose between 110 to 125 mg/dL) in the clinical setting to detect people with glucose intolerance at an earlier stage in the natural history of the disease. The presence of IFG and IGT both indicate an increased risk for other syndromes associated with insulin resistance such as hypertension and dyslipidemia that also require an aggressive diagnostic and therapeutic plan.

Understanding the natural history of type 2 diabetes aids the clinician in identifying those patients most at risk for developing diabetes and in developing an effective treatment plan for those who already have the disease. Each of the available classes of oral antidiabetic agents has a different mechanism of action and is, therefore, potentially most effective at different stages in the continuum from IGT and IFG to frank diabetes. Given that insulin resistance is the major pathogenic factor in the prediabetic state of IGT and continues to persist in frank diabetes, efforts to enhance insulin sensitivity primarily in peripheral tissues with thiazolidinedione therapy or in the liver using the biguanide metformin may be extremely useful as first-line agents in the prevention and early treatment of diabetes.

The potential benefits of intervening before the onset of diabetes and aggressive treatment once the disease becomes manifest are tremendous. Identifying and treating the individual with IGT will most likely reduce the incidence of macrovascular disease and type 2 diabetes. Early intervention in type 2 diabetes certainly reduces the incidence of microvascular disease and will most likely slow the progression of the disease itself. The primary care provider is uniquely posed to promote and provide early prevention and to have a substantial impact on lessening the burden placed on individuals and society by type 2 diabetes.

SUGGESTED READING

DeFronzo RA. The triumvirate: B-cell, muscle, liver. A collusion responsible for NIDDM. *Diabetes*. 1988;37:667-687.

DeFronzo RA, Ferrannini E. Insulin resistance. A multi-faceted syndrome responsible for NIDDM, obesity, hypertension, dyslipidemia and atherosclerotic cardiovascular disease. *Diabetes Care*. 1991;14:173-194.

Diabetes Prevention Program. Design and methods for a clinical trial in the prevention of type 2 diabetes. *Diabetes Care*. 1999;22:623-634.

Diabetes Prevention Program Research Group: Baseline characteristics of the randomized cohort. *Diabetes Care*. 2000;23:1619-1629.

Eriksson J, Franssila-Kallunki A, Ekstrand A, et al. Early metabolic defects in persons at increased risk for non–insulin-dependent diabetes mellitus. *N Engl J Med*. 1989;321:337-343.

Garvey WT, Olefsky JM, Griffin J, Hammon R, Kolterman OG. The effects of insulin treatment on insulin secretion and action in type II diabetes mellitus. *Diabetes*. 1985;34:222-234.

Granner DK, O'Brien RM. Molecular physiology and genetics of NIDDM. Importance of metabolic staging. *Diabetes Care*. 1992;15:369-395.

Haffner SM, Stern MP, Hazuda HP, Mitchell BD, Patterson JK. Cardiovascular risk factors in confirmed prediabetic individuals. Does the clock for coronary heart disease start ticking before the onset on clinical diabetes? *JAMA*. 1990;263:2893-2898.

Hamman RF. Genetic and environmental determinations of non–insulin-dependent diabetes mellitus (NIDDM). *Diabetes Metab Rev*. 1992;8:287-338.

Henry RR, Gumbiner B, Ditzler ST, Wallace P, Lyon R, Glauber HS. Intensive conventional insulin therapy for type II diabetes: metabolic effects during a 6-month outpatient trial. *Diabetes Care.* 1993;16:21-31.

Henry RR, Wallace P, Olefsky JM. Effects of weight loss on mechanisms of hyperglycemia in obese non–insulin-dependent diabetes mellitus. *Diabetes.* 1986;35:990-998.

Hu FB, Manson J, Stampfer MJ, et al. Diet, lifestyle, and the risk of type 2 diabetes mellitus in women. *N Engl J Med.* 2001;345:790-797.

Hu FB, Van Dam RM, Liu S. Diet and risk of type 2 diabetes: the role of types of fat and carbohydrate. *Diabetologia.* 2001;44:805-817.

Kobberling J, Tillil H. Genetic and nutritional factors in the etiology and pathogenesis of diabetes mellitus. *World Rev Nutr Diet.* 1990;63:102-115.

Manson JE, Ajani UA, Liu S, Nathan DM, Hennekens CH. A prospective study of cigarette smoking and the incidence of diabetes mellitus among US male physicians. *Am J Med.* 2000;109:538-542.

Olefsky JM. Etiology and pathogenesis of non–insulin-dependent diabetes (type II). In: *DeGroot: Endocrinology*, 2nd ed. New York, NY: Grune and Stratton, Inc; 1989:1369-1388.

Olefsky JM. Insulin resistance and the pathogenesis of non–insulin-dependent diabetes mellitus: cellular and molecular mechanisms. In: Efendic S, Ostenson CG, Vranic M, eds. *New Concepts in the Pathogenesis of NIDDM*. New York, NY: Plenum Publishing Corporation; 1995.

O'Rahilly S, Wainscoat JS, Turner RC. Type 2 (non–insulin-dependent) diabetes mellitus. New genetics for old nightmares. *Diabetologia.* 1988;31:407-414.

Pan XR, Li GW, Wang JX, et al. Effects of diet and exercise in preventing NIDDM in people with impaired glucose tolerance. The Da Qing IGT and Diabetes Study. *Diabetes Care.* 1997;20:537-544.

Permutt MA. Genetics of NIDDM. *Diabetes Care.* 1990; 13:1150-1153.

Ramlo-Halsted BA, Edelman SV. The natural history of type 2 diabetes. *Primary Care Clin North Am.* 1998;26:771-789.

Reaven GM. Banting lecture. Role of insulin resistance in human disease. *Diabetes.* 1988;37:1595-1607.

Rich SS. Mapping genes in diabetes: genetic epidemiological perspective. *Diabetes.* 1990;39:1315-1319.

Seely BL, Olefsky JM. Potential cellular and genetic mechanisms for insulin resistance in common disorders of obesity and diabetes. In: Moller D, ed. *Insulin Resistance and Its Clinical Disorders.* London, England: John Wiley & Sons, Ltd; 1993:187-252.

Tominaga M, Eguchi H, Manaka H, Igarashi K, Kato T, Sekikawa A. Impaired glucose tolerance is a risk factor for cardiovascular disease, but not impaired fasting glucose. The Funagata Diabetes Study. *Diabetes Care.* 1999;22:920-924.

Tuomilehto J, Lindstrom J, Eriksson JG, et al. Prevention of type 2 diabetes mellitus by changes in lifestyle among subjects with impaired glucose tolerance. *N Engl J Med.* 2001;344:1343-1350.

United Kingdom Prospective Diabetes Study Group. Overview of 6 years' therapy of type 2 diabetes: a progressive disease (UKPDS 16). *Diabetes.* 1995;44:1249-1258.

Warram JH, Martin BC, Krolewski AS, Soeldner JS, Kahn CR. Slow glucose removal rate and hyperinsulinemia precede the development of type II diabetes in the offspring of diabetic parents. *Ann Intern Med.* 1990;113:909-915.

Weyer C, Bogardus C, Moss DM, Pratley RE. The natural history of insulin secretory dysfunction and insulin resistance in the pathogenesis of type 2 diabetes mellitus. *J Clin Invest.* 1999;104:787-794.

2

3 Classification

Diabetes mellitus and other categories of glucose intolerance can be divided into three main clinical categories:

- Diabetes mellitus (with four clinical subclasses)
- Impaired glucose tolerance (IGT)
- Gestational diabetes mellitus (GDM).

The common denominator of a group of disorders that constitute the syndrome of diabetes mellitus is fasting or postprandial (random) hyperglycemia with plasma glucose levels above the limits established by the American Diabetes Association Clinical Practice Recommendations 2002. The five subclasses of diabetes mellitus are:

- Type 1 diabetes mellitus (insulin-dependent)
- Type 2 diabetes mellitus (non–insulin-dependent)
- GDM
- Malnutrition-related diabetes mellitus.
- Other types of diabetes associated with certain conditions.

Each of these subclasses has distinctive characteristics (Table 3.1).

Type 1 Diabetes Mellitus

Type 1 diabetes is defined by the presence of ketosis caused by complete or almost complete lack of insulin. Immunologic destruction of the β-cells is the etiologic basis of type 1 diabetes. An autoimmune cause is suggested by evidence of circulating antibodies to islet cells, to endogenous insulin, and/or to other antigenic components of islet cells at the time of di-

TABLE 3.1 — DISTINGUISHING CHARACTERISTICS OF DIABETES MELLITUS AND OTHER DISORDERS OF GLUCOSE INTOLERANCE

Category	Distinguishing Characteristics
Type 1 diabetes (insulin-dependent)	Any age, usually not obese, often abrupt onset, signs/symptoms usually before age 20, positive urine ketone test with hyperglycemia, insulin therapy necessary to sustain life and prevent ketoacidosis
Type 2 diabetes (non-insulin-dependent)	Usually over age 30 at diagnosis, obese, few classic symptoms, not prone to ketoacidosis unless under severe physical stress (eg, infection), exogenous insulin usually not needed to control hyperglycemia for many years
Gestational diabetes mellitus (GDM)	Onset or discovery of glucose intolerance during pregnancy
Malnutrition-related diabetes mellitus	Young age (10 to 40), usually symptomatic, not prone to ketoacidosis, most require insulin therapy

Other Types of Diabetes Mellitus Associated With Certain Conditions	
Secondary to pancreatic disease	Pancreatectomy, hemochromatosis, cystic fibrosis, chronic pancreatitis
Secondary to endocrinopathies	Cushing's syndrome, acromegaly, pheochromocytoma, primary aldosteronism, glucagonoma
Secondary to drugs and chemical agents	Certain antihypertensive drugs (thiazides, diuretics, or β-blockers), glucocorticoids, estrogen-containing preparations, nicotinic acid, phenytoin, catecholamines
Associated with insulin receptor abnormalities	Acanthosis nigricans
Associated with genetic syndromes	Lipodystrophic syndromes, muscular dystrophies, Huntington's chorea
Associated with miscellaneous conditions	Polycystic ovary disease
Impaired glucose tolerance (IGT)	Plasma glucose levels are higher after a glucose load than normal but not diagnostic of diabetes mellitus

American Diabetes Association. Clinical Practice Recommendations 2002. Report of the expert committee on the diagnosis and classification of diabetes mellitus. *Diabetes Care.* 2002;25(suppl 1):S5-S20.

3

agnosis. Patients commonly are lean and may have experienced considerable weight loss prior to diagnosis. Most are diagnosed before age 20 years, although type 1 diabetes can develop at any age. Approximately 10% of all individuals who have been diagnosed with diabetes have type 1 diabetes. Daily therapy with exogenous insulin is required throughout the patient's life to prevent metabolic decompensation, ketoacidosis, and death.

Type 2 Diabetes Mellitus

Type 2 diabetes is the most common type of diabetes, accounting for 85% to 90% of all diagnosed cases in the United States, and is more prevalent among various non-Caucasian ethnic/racial populations, such as Native Americans, African Americans, Pacific Islanders, and Hispanics. A strong genetic basis exists for type 2 diabetes (approximately 90% of patients with type 2 diabetes have a positive family history of this disorder). In addition, identical twin studies have revealed a 60% to 90% concordance for diabetes. An absence of ketosis is one of the primary features that distinguishes type 2 diabetes from type 1 diabetes, although it is possible to have ketonemia with type 2 diabetes.

Patients with type 2 diabetes can vary considerably in their ability to secrete insulin. Insulin secretion, however, is inadequate to overcome the insulin resistance associated with this type of diabetes. Defects of insulin action (insulin resistance) are typical of type 2 diabetes.

Obesity is frequently present in type 2 diabetes. Approximately 90% of people with type 2 diabetes are obese (20% over ideal body weight) and the chances of developing type 2 diabetes double for every 20% increase in body weight in susceptible individuals. However, type 2 diabetes also can develop in

32

nonobese individuals; this is more commonly observed in older patients. The incidence of type 2 diabetes increases with age and obesity in part because people tend to gain weight and especially develop central abdominal obesity as they age.

Type 2 diabetes usually is diagnosed after the age of 30, although it is being diagnosed more frequently at a younger age (eg, 20 years old) in certain ethnic groups prone to developing diabetes. The age of onset for type 2 diabetes is progressively decreasing, and now develops in adolescents and young adults as well. Initially, patients are often asymptomatic and only occasionally display the classic symptoms of hyperglycemia (polydipsia, polyuria, polyphagia, weight loss). Because type 2 diabetes can go unrecognized for many years, the early stages of microvascular disease and frank macrovascular complications may be present by the time a diagnosis is made.

Secondary/Other Types of Diabetes Mellitus

This category of diabetes mellitus is the least common and includes diabetes related to certain other diseases, conditions, or drugs. Hyperglycemia is present at a level that is diagnostic of diabetes. Patients are placed in this category if their diabetes has a known or probable cause or is part of a specific condition or syndrome (Table 3.1). Treatment of the underlying disorder may ameliorate the diabetes; more frequently, however, it is necessary to treat the diabetes with lifestyle modifications, such as diet and exercise, and medication.

Malnutrition-Related Diabetes Mellitus

This type of diabetes is seen for the most part in developing countries and tends to affect young individuals between 10 and 40 years old. The classic symptoms of hyperglycemia are present without ketoacidosis, and insulin usually is required to control hyperglycemia. The role of malnutrition as a causal factor is unknown.

Impaired Glucose Tolerance

Individuals who have postprandial plasma glucose levels that are higher than normal but lower than established diagnostic values for diabetes mellitus are classified as having IGT (diagnostic criteria in Table 3.2). This condition is common (approximately 5% to 7% of the US population) and considered a precursor of type 2 diabetes. Although individuals with IGT are more likely to eventually develop diabetes mellitus,

---

TABLE 3.2 — DIAGNOSTIC CRITERIA FOR IMPAIRED FASTING GLUCOSE AND IMPAIRED GLUCOSE TOLERANCE USING THE ORAL GLUCOSE TOLERANCE TEST*

World Health Organization/American Diabetes Association **criteria**	
IFG	≥110 – <126 mg/dL
IGT	
Fasting	<126 mg/dL
and 2-h	≥140 – <200 mg/dL
Diabetes	
Fasting	≥126 mg/dL
and 2-h	≥200 mg/dL

Abbreviations: IFG, impaired fasting glucose; IGT, impaired glucose tolerance.

* 75-g glucose load.

American Diabetes Association. Clinical practice recommendations 2002. *Diabetes Care*. 2002;25(suppl 1).

---

only approximately 25% do develop type 2 diabetes and a similar percentage subsequently have normal glucose levels. The rate of progression is approximately 5% to 10% per year and can be influenced by:

- Ethnic origin
- Degree of obesity
- Distribution of body fat
- Sedentary lifestyle
- Aging
- Concomitant medical conditions.

Individuals with IGT are more susceptible to macrovascular disease (coronary artery, peripheral vascular, cerebrovascular), which often is present at the time of diagnosis. Pharmacologic therapies and nonpharmacologic interventions such as weight reduction, improved diet, and increased physical activity through lifestyle modifications, have been shown to prevent the progression of IGT to type 2 diabetes (see Chapter 7, *Diabetes Prevention* section).

Impaired Fasting Glucose

The American Diabetes Association (ADA) introduced a new diagnostic category called impaired fasting glucose (IFG), which is defined as an individual who has a fasting glucose value of between 110 and 125 mg/dL. This new IFG classification has major clinical implications because it allows for the earlier identification and eventual treatment of people who have undiagnosed diabetes and IGT. Individuals with IFG need to be investigated further for the cardiovascular risk factors associated with diabetes and followed closely. In addition, nonpharmacologic therapies should be instituted early, such as diet, exercise, and lifestyle modification.

Gestational Diabetes Mellitus

Glucose intolerance that is first detected during pregnancy is classified as GDM. Excluded from this group are women who had diabetes before conception. GDM occurs in about 2% to 4% of pregnant women, usually during the second or third trimester, and is more common in women who are older, obese, of high-risk ethnic groups, or have a family history of diabetes. This condition is important to identify because of the increased risk of fetal morbidity and mortality with GDM. Pregnant women of average risk should be screened with a 50-g, 1-hour glucose tolerance test during the 24th to 28th weeks of pregnancy. Women at high risk of GDM should undergo glucose testing as soon as possible. Approximately 81% to 94% of women with GDM return to normal glucose tolerance after delivery. However, women who have had GDM are at increased risk of developing type 2 diabetes, with approximately 30% to 40% developing type 2 diabetes or IGT within 10 to 20 years.

Problems With Classification

Sometimes it is difficult to distinguish between type 1 and type 2 diabetes. For example, younger type 2 patients who are thin and taking insulin may resemble type 1 patients. In addition, some patients display the characteristics of type 2 diabetes and are not susceptible to ketoacidosis, yet they are taking insulin. These patients should not be classified as type 1 based solely on their insulin regimen, because they are taking insulin for glycemic control rather than as a life-sustaining therapy to prevent ketoacidosis and death.

Type 2 diabetes sometimes is found in children or adolescents who usually are above their ideal body weight and a member of a high-risk ethnic group susceptible to type 2 diabetes. A unique type of diabetes found in the pediatric and young adult population is called maturity-onset diabetes of the young (MODY) and is an example of an autosomal dominant form of inheritance of diabetes. Age alone should not be considered the diagnostic variable in these patients; they should be classified as having type 2 and not type 1 diabetes.

Another classification problem that can occur involves older patients who develop ketosis-prone, type 1 diabetes. The onset of this form of diabetes is slower in older adults and may resemble type 2 diabetes for a considerable length of time. These individuals tend to be at or slightly below their ideal weight and respond poorly to oral antidiabetic agents. The appearance of ketones in their urine may indicate a true lack of insulin. The insulin requirements thus become obvious and insulin therapy must be started to avoid severe ketoacidosis, coma, and death. These patients tend to be more insulin sensitive than their obese counterparts with type 2 diabetes and require less insulin to control their diabetes. A positive blood test for glutamic acid decarboxylase (GAD) antibodies is indicative of type 1 diabetes.

SUGGESTED READING

American Diabetes Association. Clinical practice recommendations 2002. *Diabetes Care*. 2002;25(suppl 1).

American Diabetes Association. *Diabetes 2002 Vital Statistics*. Alexandria, Va: American Diabetes Association; 2002.

Porte D, Sherwin RS. *Ellenberg & Rifkin's Diabetes Mellitus*. 5th ed. Stamford, Conn: Appleton & Lange; 1997.

4

Diagnosis of Diabetes and the Metabolic Syndrome

A diagnosis of diabetes can be suspected in the presence of the following signs and symptoms of hyperglycemia:

- Polydipsia (increased thirst)
- Polyuria (increased urinary frequency with increased volume)
- Fatigue
- Polyphagia (increased appetite)
- Weight loss
- Abnormal healing
- Blurred vision
- Increased occurrence of infections, particularly those caused by yeast.

Only a minority of adults who are diagnosed with diabetes are symptomatic initially. Consequently, the onset of type 2 diabetes may occur years before a diagnosis is made. Individuals who are asymptomatic tend to be diagnosed during a routine physical examination, treatment for another condition, or through specific diabetes screening. The risk of diabetes is increased in asymptomatic individuals if any of the following risk factors are present:

- A strong family history of diabetes (first-degree relatives)
- Obesity (body mass index [BMI] $\geq$25 kg/m^2), particularly central adiposity
- Certain races (American Indian, Hispanic, African, Asian, or Pacific Islander ancestry)
- Women with previous gestational diabetes or history of babies of 9 pounds or more at birth

- Previously identified impaired fasting glucose (IFT) or impaired glucose tolerance (IGT)
- High-density lipoprotein (HDL) cholesterol ≤35 mg/dL and/or triglycerides ≥250 mg/dL
- Hypertension (≥140/90 mm Hg)
- 40 years of age with any of the preceding factors

Measuring plasma glucose concentrations is currently the only way to confirm a diagnosis of diabetes. Normal plasma glucose values are presented in Table 4.1 and the criteria for diagnosing diabetes in nonpregnant adults are shown in Table 4.2.

TABLE 4.1 — NORMAL PLASMA GLUCOSE VALUES FOR NONPREGNANT ADULTS		
Fasting	Time zero	<110 mg/dL (6.1 mM)
After 75-g oral glucose load	120 min	<140 mg/dL (7.8 mM)
American Diabetes Association. Clinical practice recommendations 2002. *Diabetes Care*. 2002;25(suppl 1).		

Three approaches to glucose testing can be used to diagnose diabetes:
- Fasting plasma glucose measurements
- Random plasma glucose measurements
- Oral glucose tolerance testing (OGTT).

The fasting plasma glucose test is the diagnostic test of choice and is used to diagnose approximately 90% of all individuals with type 2 diabetes. Plasma glucose testing may be performed in individuals who have had food or beverages shortly before the test. This type of testing is referred to as random plasma glucose testing. An OGTT measuring only the fasting and 2-hour blood glucose can give excellent diagnostic data and is fairly easy to perform. Because the glycosylated he-

TABLE 4.2 — CRITERIA FOR THE DIAGNOSIS OF DIABETES MELLITUS

One or more of the following must be present:

- Symptoms of diabetes plus casual plasma glucose concentration ≥200 mg/dL (11.1 mmol/L). Casual is defined as any time of day without regard to time since last meal. The classic symptoms of diabetes include:
  - Polyuria
  - Polydipsia
  - Unexplained weight loss
- Fasting plasma glucose (FPG) ≥126 mg/dL (7.0 mmol/L). Fasting is defined as no caloric intake for at least 8 hours
- Two-hour postload glucose (PG) ≥200 mg/dL (11.1 mmol/L) during an oral glucose tolerance test (OGTT). The test should be performed as described by the World Health Organization (WHO), using a glucose load containing the equivalent of 75-g anhydrous glucose dissolved in water

In the absence of unequivocal hyperglycemia with acute metabolic decompensation, these criteria should be confirmed by repeat testing on a different day. The third measure (OGTT) is not recommended for routine clinical use.

American Diabetes Association. Clinical practice recommendations 2002. Report of the expert committee on the diagnosis and classification of diabetes mellitus. *Diabetes Care*. 2002;25(suppl 1):S5-S20.

moglobin test has not been standardized, it is not currently used for diagnosing diabetes.

Regardless of the type of test used, all abnormal laboratory values should be documented at least twice to avoid a misdiagnosis caused by laboratory errors, unless all values are extremely high or classic symptoms are present. An OGTT generally is not necessary for diagnosing diabetes. However, an OGTT can be useful for evaluating high-risk individuals so that preventive measures can be started (diet modification, exercise, weight loss) at an early stage. The American Diabetes Association and the World Health Organization (WHO) have prepared criteria for diagnosing diabetes mellitus and IGT based on the OGTT (Table 3.2).

In the absence of an elevated fasting glucose ($\geq$126 mg/dL) or a casual plasma glucose of >200 mg/dL (confirmed on a subsequent day), pregnant women should undergo risk assessment for gestational diabetes at the first prenatal visit. Women at low risk of developing glucose intolerance during pregnancy need not be tested for gestational diabetes. Women at high risk (marked obesity, previous history of gestational diabetes, glycosuria, high-risk racial/ethnic groups, or strong family history of diabetes) should undergo glucose testing as soon as possible. Testing involves a 50-g glucose load without regard to the time of the last meal or the time of day. If not found to have gestational diabetes at initial screening, retesting should be conducted during the 24th to 28th week of gestation. This test is only recommended in individuals at risk for diabetes. A 1-hour plasma glucose concentration of >130 mg/dL is considered a positive reading that calls for a formal OGTT with a 100-g glucose load and sampling at fasting 1, 2, and 3 hours after glucose challenge. The diagnosis of gestational diabetes is made when two or more of these samples meet or exceed the following values: fasting, 95 mg/dL; 1-hour, 180 mg/dL; 2-hour, 155 mg/dL; and 3-hour, 140 mg/dL.

A complete medical evaluation is indicated following a positive diagnostic blood test for diabetes. Patients should not be diagnosed on the basis of age alone. The purpose of this evaluation is to:
- Appropriately classify the patient
- Detect any underlying diseases that may require further evaluation

- Determine whether any of the complications of diabetes are present.

Figure 4.1 shows a Diabetes Warranty Program developed as a reference for patients, outlining evaluations at every visit and annually. Getting patients involved in their own care is an important tool to improve compliance and motivation.

Diabetes and Cardiovascular Disease Risk Assessment

4

Diabetes is now recognized as a cardiovascular disease equivalent. That is, an individual with diabetes but without evidence of overt heart disease has the same risk of a myocardial infarction (MI) as a nondiabetic individual who has had a previous cardiovascular event. Diabetes is an independent risk factor for cardiovascular disease in both men and women. Women lose the protective effect against cardiovascular disease when they develop diabetes. Two of every three people with diabetes die of cardiovascular disease. Once a person with diabetes develops clinical evidence of cardiovascular disease, their likelihood of survival is worse than that of nondiabetics with cardiovascular disease.

Most patients with type 2 diabetes have tissue resistance to insulin. The presence of insulin resistance is associated with and predisposes to both cardiovascular disease and type 2 diabetes. Like type 2 diabetes, insulin resistance is influenced by genetic susceptibility, obesity, physical inactivity, and advancing age. Patients with insulin resistance tend to develop the metabolic or dysmetabolic syndrome. This is associated with:
- Abdominal obesity
- Atherogenic dyslipidemia
- Hypertension

FIGURE 4.1 — DIABETES WARRANTY PROGRAM

What Should Be Done at *Every Visit* (3-6 months)

	Date	Result	Normal Range or Goal
Weight			
Blood pressure (sitting and standing)			
Foot examination*			
Glycosylated hemoglobin or fructosamine[†] (know the normal range)			

What Tests/Examinations Should Be Done at Least *Every Year*

	Date	Result (recommendations)	Normal Range
Cholesterol levels (fasting):			
• Total cholesterol			
• Triglycerides			
• HDL			
• LDL			

Urine protein (microalbumin)					
Serum creatinine					
Thyroid function test (TSH)					
Eye examination (dilated)					
Dental examination					
Other tests/examinations (depending on individual needs):					
•Cardiologist (for heart disease)					
•Podiatrist (for foot problems)					
•Gastroenterologist (for stomach problems)					

* Visual, tuning fork, 10-g monofilament, palpitation.
† Glycosylated hemoglobin and fructosamine are long-term diabetes control factors.

Source: Edelman SV. Diabetes Warranty Program. VA Endocrinology Clinic, VA Hospital, UCSD, La Jolla, California.

- Glucose intolerance
- A procoagulant state
- Evidence of vascular inflammation.

Recently, the National Cholesterol Education Program (NCEP) published guidelines on detection, evaluation, and treatment of high blood cholesterol in adults (Adult Treatment Panel III). These guidelines are based on clinical trial data and other scientific rationale.

The new NCEP guidelines emphasize multiple risk factors (two or more) in its primary-prevention strategy. The primary target of therapy and a major cause of coronary heart disease (CHD) is low-density lipoprotein (LDL) cholesterol. Numerous recent clinical trials clearly demonstrate LDL-cholesterol lowering reduces risk for CHD, even in individuals with type 2 diabetes. The NCEP advocates that the intensity of risk-reduction therapy or primary prevention of CHD be adjusted based on an individuals's absolute risk. Majors risk factors include:

- High LDL cholesterol
- Cigarette smoking
- Hypertension $\geq$140/90 mm Hg or patient on antihypertensive therapy
- Low high-density lipoprotein (HDL) cholesterol (<40 mg/dL)
- Family history of premature heart disease (<55 years in male first-degree relative, <65 years in female first-degree relative)
- Advancing age: $\geq$45 years of age in men, and $\geq$55 years of age in women.

Diabetes is considered as a CHD risk equivalent and therefore a major risk factor. An HDL cholesterol level $\geq$60 mg/dL represents a negative risk factor and negates one positive risk factor from the total count.

The NCEP guidelines establish the goal of an LDL level <100 mg/dL when CHD or a risk equivalent such as diabetes is present. The American Diabetes Association has established similar guidelines, including an order of priorities for the treatment of diabetic dyslipidemia in adults. After LDL cholesterol lowering follows HDL cholesterol raising, triglyceride lowering, and treatment of combined hyperlipidemia.

The Metabolic or Dysmetabolic Syndrome

The NCEP guidelines recently recognized the metabolic syndrome as a secondary target of risk-reduction therapy after LDL cholesterol lowering, which is the primary target. The constellation of abnormalities that constitute the metabolic syndrome enhance the risk for CHD at any given LDL level. By the NCEP criteria, the diagnosis of the metabolic syndrome requires three or more of the risk determinants shown in Table 4.3. Most individuals with type 2 diabetes have multiple risk determinants of the metabolic syndrome. First-line therapy for all components of the metabolic syndrome involves weight reduction/control and increased physical activity. Other components of the syndrome (high triglyceride levels, low HDL-cholesterol levels, dyslipidemia, glucose intolerance, a procoagulant state, and hypertension) may require specific pharmacologic management to achieve adequate control.

Most individuals with type 2 diabetes and components of the metabolic syndrome usually receive:

- An angiotensin-converting enzyme (ACE) inhibitor and/or an angiotensin II receptor blocker (ARB) as initial therapy for hypertension and/or microalbuminuria

TABLE 4.3 — CLINICAL CRITERIA OF THE METABOLIC SYNDROME*	
Risk Factor	**Defining Level**
Abdominal obesity (waist circumference)	Men >40 inches (102 cm)
	Women >35 inches (88 cm)
Triglycerides	≥150 mg/dL
HDL cholesterol	Men <40 mg/dL
	Women <50 mg/dL
Blood pressure	≥130/ ≥85 mm Hg
Fasting glucose	>110 mg/dL
Abbreviation: HDL, high-density lipoprotein.	
* Metabolic Syndrome is synonymous to the Dysmetabolic Syndrome X or Insulin Resistance Syndrome.	
JAMA. 2001;285:2486-2497.	

- Enteric-coated aspirin at doses of 81 to 325 mg/day to reduce the prothrombotic or procoagulant state
- An HMG-CoA reductase inhibitor to reduce LDL cholesterol to <100 mg/dL, together with specific therapy for hyperglycemia and other possible risk determinants.

The Centers for Disease Control (CDC) recently recognized the Metabolic or Dysmetabolic Syndrome X with a new ICD-9-CM code of 277.7. The CDC does not require that a given number of components be present to use this ICD-9 code, but instead relies on the professional opinion of the physician that the Dysmetabolic Syndrome X is present. The American Association of Clinical Endocrinologists (AACE) has suggested major and minor criteria to assist physicians

TABLE 4.4 — MAJOR AND MINOR CRITERIA FOR THE DYSMETABOLIC SYNDROME X*

Major Criteria
- Insulin resistance (denoted by hyperinsulinemia relative to glucose levels)
- Acanthosis nigricans
- Central obesity (waist circumference >102 cm for men and >88 cm for women)
- Dyslipidemia (HDL <45 mg/dL for women; <35 mg/dL for men, or triglycerides >150 mg/dL)
- Hypertension
- Impaired fasting glucose or type 2 diabetes
- Hyperuricemia

Minor Criteria
- Hypercoagulability
- Polycystic ovary syndrome
- Vascular endothelial dysfunction
- Microalbuminuria
- Coronary heart disease

* Criteria developed by the American Association of Clinical Endocrinologists.

in making the diagnosis. These are show in Table 4.4. Many of the criteria advocated by AACE are similar to those of the NCEP guidelines.

SUGGESTED READING

American Diabetes Association. Clinical practice recommendations 2002. *Diabetes Care*. 2002;25(suppl 1).

American Diabetes Association. *Diabetes 2002 Vital Statistics*. Alexandria, Va: American Diabetes Association; 2002.

Porte D, Sherwin RS. *Ellenberg & Rifkin's Diabetes Mellitus*. 5th ed. Stamford, Conn: Appleton & Lange; 1997.

Edelman SV. *Taking Control of Your Diabetes*. 2nd ed. Professional Communications: Caddo, OK; 2001.

Executive Summary of the Third Report of the National Cholesterol Education Program (NCEP) Expert Panel on Detection, Evaluation, and Treatment of High Blood Cholesterol in Adults (Adult Treatment Panel III). *JAMA*. 2001;285:2486-2497.

5   Nutrition

Nutrition Therapy

One of the most fundamental components of the diabetes treatment plan for all patients with type 2 diabetes is nutrition therapy. Specific goals of nutrition therapy in type 2 diabetes are to:

- Achieve and maintain as near-normal blood glucose levels as possible by balancing food intake with physical activity, supplemented by oral hypoglycemic agents and/or insulin as needed
- Normalize blood pressure
- Normalize serum lipid levels
- Help patients attain and maintain a reasonable body weight (defined as the weight an individual and healthcare provider acknowledge as possible to achieve and maintain on a short- and long-term basis)
- Promote overall health through optimal nutrition and lifestyle behaviors.

Because no single dietary approach is appropriate for all patients and given the heterogeneous nature of type 2 diabetes, meal plans and diet modifications should be individualized to meet a patient's unique needs and lifestyle. Accordingly, any nutrition intervention should be based on a thorough assessment of a patient's typical food intake and eating habits and should include an evaluation of current nutritional status.

Some patients with mild-to-moderate diabetes can be effectively treated with an appropriate balance of diet modification and exercise as the sole therapeutic intervention, particularly if their fasting blood glucose level is <140 mg/dL. The majority of patients, however, will require pharmacologic intervention in addition to diet and exercise prescriptions. It is important to note that pharmacologic treatment is often less successful when the patient is not on some type of dietary and exercise regimen.

Dietary changes do not have to be dramatic to produce clinically important results in terms of improving blood glucose, blood pressure, and lipid levels. Regular monitoring of blood glucose, glycated hemoglobin, lipid levels, blood pressure, and body weight serves as an ongoing assessment of the nutrition intervention.

Nutrition Consult

Because nutrition issues and meal planning are complex, a registered dietitian who is familiar with the current principles and recommendations for managing diabetes may be consulted after a patient is diagnosed with diabetes. This healthcare professional can be an essential member of the diabetes management team and performs a number of valuable functions:

- Conducts initial assessment of nutritional status:
  - Diet history
  - Lifestyle
  - Eating habits
- Provides patient education regarding:
  - The basic principles of diet therapy for diabetes
  - Meal planning
  - Problem-solving techniques for changing eating behaviors
- Develops an individualized meal plan:
  - Emphasizing one or two priorities

- Minimizing changes from the patient's usual diet (to encourage compliance)
- Provides follow-up assessment of the meal plan to:
  - Determine effectiveness in terms of glucose and lipid control and weight loss
  - Make necessary changes based on weight loss, activity level, or changes in medication
- Provides ongoing patient education and support (particularly for those on weight-loss regimens), helping patients learn to adjust their meal plans for various situations.

Body Weight Considerations 5

Weight loss frequently is a primary goal of nutrition therapy because 80% to 90% of people with type 2 diabetes are obese. Caloric restriction and weight loss, even as small as 5 lb in body weight, can result in:

- Improved glucose control
- Increased sensitivity to insulin
- Improved lipid levels and blood pressure
- The need for a corresponding lowering of the dosage of pharmacologic agents (eg, oral antidiabetic medications and insulin).

Weight loss is associated with improved glucose uptake and insulin sensitivity as well as decreased hepatic glucose production. Consequently, the therapeutic regimen most useful for individuals with obesity and glucose intolerance is weight reduction via nutrition therapy and increased physical activity. If moderate weight loss does not improve metabolic parameters, however, pharmacologic therapy (oral antidiabetic agents or insulin) may need to be added to the regimen.

Weight loss and subsequent weight maintenance can be one of the most difficult and challenging aspects of managing diabetes. Therefore, emphasis should be placed on achieving and maintaining normal blood glucose control as the goal of nutrition therapy, using nutritionally balanced meal plans that promote gradual weight loss as a means to achieve this metabolic goal. A reasonable approach that provides a combination of the following strategies increases the chances of a successful outcome:

- Modest caloric restriction
- Restriction of saturated fat intake
- Spreading caloric intake throughout the day
- Increased physical activity
- Behavior modification techniques for changing eating habits and attitudes and promoting healthy, long-term lifestyle behaviors
- Psychosocial support.

Suggested weights for adults based on the USDA *Dietary Guidelines for Americans* (1990) are shown in Table 5.1. The upper end of the ranges are considered appropriate weights for men, given their greater bone and muscle mass; the lower end of the ranges are for women, who have comparatively less bone and muscle mass.

Approximately 10% of patients with type 2 diabetes are of normal weight and do not need to restrict their caloric intake. For these individuals, nutrition therapy focuses on distributing calorie as well as nutrient intake and content throughout the day to achieve optimal glucose, lipid, and blood pressure control. The pattern of spreading out calories and carbohydrates between meals and snacks is individualized based on results of self-monitoring of blood glucose.

TABLE 5.1 — SUGGESTED WEIGHT FOR ADULTS

Height	Weight (lb)	
	19 - 34 (yr)	≥ 35 (yr)
5' 0"	97-128	108-138
5' 1"	101-132	111-143
5' 2"	104-137	115-148
5' 3"	107-141	119-152
5' 4"	111-146	122-157
5' 5"	114-150	126-162
5' 6"	118-155	130-167
5' 7"	121-160	134-172
5' 8"	125-164	138-178
5' 9"	129-169	142-183
5'10"	132-174	146-188
5'11"	136-179	151-194
6' 0"	140-184	155-199
6' 1"	144-189	159-205
6' 2"	148-195	164-210
6' 3"	152-200	168-216
6' 4"	156-205	173-222
6' 5"	160-211	173-222
6' 6"	164-216	182-234

US Department of Agriculture. US Department of Health and Human Services. *Nutrition and Your Health: Dietary Guidelines for Americans*, 3rd ed. Hyattsville, Md: USDA Human Nutrition Information Service; 1990.

5

Calorie Intake

Adult calorie needs vary according to age, activity level, and desired weight change. The following formula can be used to determine adult calorie requirements. First calculate desired body weight:

- Women: 100 lb for the first 5 ft of height plus 5 lb for each additional inch over 5 ft
- Men: 106 lb for the first 5 ft of height plus 6 lb for each additional inch over 5 ft
- Add 10% for larger body builds; subtract 10% for smaller body builds.

Then, multiply the resulting weight by one of the following to compute calorie need based on desired weight:

- Men and physically active women: multiply by 15
- Most women, sedentary men, and adults over age 55: multiply by 13
- Sedentary women, obese adults, sedentary adults over age 55: multiply by 10.

If weight loss is indicated, daily calorie intake needs to be adjusted to produce the necessary deficit. Given that a 3500-calorie deficit per week is required to produce a 1-pound loss of fat, a decrease of approximately 500 to 1000 calories per day is needed to lose 1 to 2 pounds of fat per week. Regular exercise is an excellent way to create a calorie deficit and has been associated with successful weight maintenance. Because calorie restriction alone can be difficult to maintain, some people have greater success by eliminating 250 to 500 calories from their daily diet and increasing daily activity by 250 to 500 calories.

Nutrient Composition of the Diet

A nutritionally balanced diet is as important for individuals with diabetes as for nondiabetics. Diet prescriptions for those with type 2 diabetes need to take into account the higher prevalence of dyslipidemia, atherosclerosis, and hypertension in this population. Practical dietary recommendations are outlined in Table 5.2.

■ **Protein Intake**

The Recommended Dietary Allowance (RDA) for adults as advised by the USDA is used as the guideline for protein intake for patients with type 2 diabetes (0.8 g/kg body weight/day). This equates to a small-to-medium portion of protein once daily with either breakfast, lunch, or dinner. Protein allowance therefore amounts to 15% to 20% of daily calories and should be derived from both animal and vegetable sources. Vegetable protein may be less nephrotoxic than animal protein and thus restriction of vegetable protein may not be necessary. In following these recommendations, meat, fish, or poultry consumption would need to be limited to 3 to 5 oz daily.

The long-term consequences of high-protein (>30% of total daily calories) and low-carbohydrate diets are unknown, but may aggravate renal impairment in diabetic individuals. High-protein diets are often high in saturated fats which have an adverse effect on LDL cholesterol.

Because excessive protein intake may aggravate renal insufficiency, type 2 patients with evidence of overt nephropathy should be encouraged to limit their protein intake to approximately 10% of daily calories or ≤0.8 g/kg body weight/day. In short-term studies, more severe restriction of protein (0.6 g/kg body weight/day) has been shown to be effective in slowing the progression of kidney disease in patients with

TABLE 5.2 — PRACTICAL DIETARY RECOMMENDATIONS

- Emphasize to the obese diabetic patient that even small amounts of weight loss can have substantial benefits on glucose, lipids, and blood pressure levels. Weight reduction should be constantly encouraged through lifestyle modification since the natural course with diabetes is to gain weight
- Sugar (sucrose) and sugar-containing foods do not increase blood glucose levels any greater than equivalent amounts of starch and do not need to be restricted. They can be substituted for other carbohydrate sources in the context of a healthy diet
- When intensive insulin therapy is used, premeal insulin doses should be adjusted based on the carbohydrate content of the meal (carbohydrate counting). A rough guide is approximately 1 unit of insulin for every 15 g carbohydrate, but it should be individualized
- When on a fixed daily insulin dose, day-to-day carbohydrate intake should be as consistent as possible.
- All fats are calorie-dense and contribute to weight gain when consumed in excess. Not all fats are created equal. Monounsaturated fat (eg, olive oil) and polyunsaturated fats including fish oil (N-3 polyunsaturated fatty acids) have beneficial effects on lipid levels and may exert cardioprotective benefit
- Saturated (animal-derived) fats and transunsaturated fatty acids (processed hydrogenated vegetable oils) have detrimental effects on lipids and should be avoided as much as possible. This is best achieved by limiting intake of red meat, cheese, and whole milk
- Exercise of any form is beneficial and more effective when regular and sustained. As little as 30 minutes five times per week is helpful in losing or maintaining weight, lowering glucose and blood pressure, and improving lipid profiles
- Moderate alcohol intake can reduce cardiovascular risk, but should be limited to one drink for adult women and two drinks for adult men daily consumed with food. One drink is equivalent to 12 oz of beer, 5 oz of wine, or 1.5 oz of distilled spirits

> - High-salt intake contributes to hypertension (high blood pressure) and should be limited to that usually found in food. Patients should be encouraged not to eat processed meats, salty snacks, or add salt to food.
> - Unless there is evidence of deficiency, vitamin, anti-oxidant, and mineral supplementation is generally not necessary. Folic acid supplements have benefit to prevent birth defects and calcium to prevent osteoporosis

diabetes who already have some renal insufficiency. However, severely restricted protein diets have also been reported to be associated with loss of muscle mass and strength. Evidence exists that a low-protein diet can reverse the rate of deterioration in renal function.

■ Fat Intake

The remaining 80% to 85% of daily calories are distributed between fat and carbohydrate intake, based on a patient's nutrition assessment and treatment goals (glucose, lipid, and weight outcomes). Several important benefits support the restriction of dietary fat in patients with type 2 diabetes:

- Excess consumption of dietary fat may contribute to obesity, which is common in the majority of patients with type 2 diabetes. Restricting dietary fat may limit the development or reduce the extent of obesity.
- Abnormal lipid levels often are associated with both obesity and diabetes and increase the risk of cardiovascular disease. Reduced intake of saturated fat can have beneficial effects by reducing triglyceride and low-density lipoprotein (LDL) cholesterol, and increasing high-density lipoprotein (HDL) cholesterol.

Therefore, the following guidelines are recommended for fat intake to promote weight loss, achieve lipid goals, and reduce cardiovascular risk:

- Reduce dietary fat to <30% of total calories
- Limit saturated fat to <10% of total calories, and <7% of calories in patients with elevated LDL cholesterol
- Limit polyunsaturated fats to 10% of total calories
- Limit daily cholesterol consumption to 300 mg; limit to <200 mg/day if lipids are elevated
- Moderately increase intake of monounsaturated fats such as canola and olive oil (up to 20% of calories). A diet high in monounsaturated fats has been shown to improve glucose control, lower triglycerides, and raise HDL levels.

Effectiveness of dietary fat modification is determined by regular monitoring of glycemic control, triglyceride and cholesterol status, and body weight, with periodic adjustments based on metabolic response to the diet.

■ Carbohydrate Intake

The carbohydrate allowance is determined after protein and fat intake have been calculated and is individualized based on eating habits and glucose and lipid goals. Emphasis is placed on whole grains, starches, fruits, and vegetables to provide the necessary vitamins, minerals, and fiber in the diet. The recommended daily consumption of fiber is the same for people with diabetes as for nondiabetics (20 g to 35 g). Although dietary fiber can improve serum lipid levels, the effect on glycemic control is modest at best.

Traditionally, complex carbohydrates were thought to produce lower blood glucose responses than simple sugars because sugars are digested and absorbed more rapidly. This belief, which influenced previous recommendations of replacing simple sugars in the diet with complex carbohydrates, has been largely disproved by clinical research. For example, the glycemic response to fruits and milk has been found to be lower than the response to most starches, and sucrose has been found to produce a glycemic response similar to that of bread, rice, and potatoes. The rate of digestion of a given food seems to be more related to the presence of fat, degree of ripeness, cooking method, form, and preparation.

■ Sucrose

A modest amount of sugar is allowed in the daily diet of patients with type 2 diabetes. Sucrose and sucrose-containing foods may be substituted for other carbohydrates in the meal plan, but not simply added. Patients need to be taught how to make such substitutions using self-monitoring of blood glucose (SMBG) to evaluate the glycemic response. The total nutrient content of the sucrose-containing food should be considered, particularly because sugar and fat are the main ingredients in many sweets. Obese individuals usually are advised to avoid sweets because of the potential of a small portion triggering overconsumption.

■ Fructose

A natural source of dietary fructose is fruits and vegetables. In addition, some sweeteners are derived from these sources. Moderate consumption is recommended, particularly concerning foods in which fructose is used as a sweetening agent. Although fructose has a lower glycemic effect than sucrose, it contains the same amount of calories and therefore should be limited in hypocaloric diets. People with dyslipidemia also are advised to limit their consumption of fructose because of the potential adverse effects on serum triglyceride and LDL cholesterol levels.

■ Other Nutritive/Nonnutritive Sweeteners and Fat Substitutes

Nutritive sweeteners such as corn syrup, fruit juice/concentrate, honey, molasses, dextrose, and maltose do not seem to have a greater advantage or disadvantage over sucrose in terms of impact on calorie content or glycemic response, but they need to be accounted for in the meal plan. Certain sugar alcohols (sorbitol, mannitol, xylitol) that are commonly used as sweeteners can produce a lower glycemic response than sucrose but seem to have no real advantage over sucrose or other nutritive sweeteners when consumed as part of mixed meals. Excessive consumption of sugar alcohols may cause laxative effects.

Nonnutritive sweeteners (saccharin, aspartame, acesulfame K, sucralose) have been approved by the Food and Drug Administration (FDA) for consumption by people with diabetes. These sweeteners are useful because they contribute minimal or no calories or carbohydrates to the diet when they are used as tabletop sweeteners or in soft drinks. However, when sweeteners are used in foods that contain other nutrients and calories (ice cream, cookies, puddings), the foods must be worked into the meal plan or consult with a nutritionist.

Because many of the fat substitutes, such as Olestra, currently being used are derived from carbohydrate or protein sources, the content of these compounds is increased above the usual amounts in such products. Patients need to be advised to review the carbohydrate and/or protein content when using products with fat substitutes.

■ Vitamins, Minerals, and Herbs

Supplementation generally is not recommended for people with diabetes when dietary intake is adequate and balanced. Patients who become chromium-deficient as a result of long-term parenteral nutrition may require chromium supplementation. However, most people with diabetes are not chromium-deficient and do not benefit from supplementation. Similarly, magnesium does not need to be added to the diets of most patients with diabetes unless routine evaluation of serum magnesium reveals a deficiency. Patients taking diuretics may need potassium supplementation. However, hyperkalemia may require potassium restriction in patients with renal insufficiency, or hyporeninemic hypoaldosteronism, or in those taking angiotensin-converting enzyme (ACE) inhibitors. One consideration may be the potential value of antioxidant supplements (vitamin C and beta-carotene) in reducing atherosclerotic lesions and cataracts, both of which are common in type 2 diabetes. The value of such supplementation is yet to be confirmed.

There are many nonprescription herbal remedies being touted in health food stores as being beneficial for people with diabetes. While some of these herbs may have some rational scientific basis, most have not been well studied and the benefits are questionable. Some of these compounds have the potential to produce toxicity.

■ **Alcohol Intake**

The same recommendations used for the general population are appropriate for people with type 2 diabetes. Moderate consumption will not adversely affect blood glucose in patients whose diabetes is well controlled. Calories from alcohol should be included as part of the total calorie intake and reflected in the meal plan as a substitute for fat (one alcoholic beverage = two fat exchanges). For patients taking insulin, one or two alcoholic beverages per day are acceptable (one alcoholic beverage = 12 oz beer, 5 oz wine, or 1½ oz distilled spirits; sweet drinks should be avoided) taken with or in addition to the meal plan. However, some special considerations exist regarding alcohol intake. Patients taking insulin or sulfonylureas are susceptible to hypoglycemia if alcohol is consumed on an empty stomach. Therefore, these individuals should make sure to take any desired alcohol with a meal and perform frequent home glucose monitoring.

SUGGESTED READING

American Diabetes Association. Clinical practice recommendations 2002. Evidence-based nutrition principles and recommendations for the treatment and prevention of diabetes and related complications. *Diabetes Care*. 2002;25(suppl 1);S50-S60.

American Diabetes Association. *Medical Management of Non–insulin-dependent (Type II) Diabetes,* 3rd ed. Alexandria, Va: American Diabetes Association; 1994:22-39.

Henry RR. Protein content of the diabetic diet. *Diabetes Care*. 1994;17:1502-1513.

Mudaliar SR, Henry RR. Role of glycemic control and protein restriction in clinical management of diabetic kidney disease. *Endocr Pract*. 1996;2:220-226.

Porte D, Sherwin RS. *Ellenburg & Rifkin's Diabetes Mellitus*. 5th ed. Stamford, Conn: Appleton & Lange; 1997.

6   Exercise

Many adults with diabetes are sedentary and obese, which can contribute to the development of glucose intolerance. Therefore, physical activity should be included as an essential treatment component in the diabetes management plan unless contraindicated in a given individual. Current research suggests that even low-level regular exercise can prevent or delay the onset of type 2 diabetes in susceptible, high-risk individuals.

Benefits

The potential benefits of regular exercise include:
- Improved glucose tolerance because of enhanced insulin sensitivity
- Weight loss or maintenance of a desirable body weight because of increased energy expenditure
- Improved cardiovascular risk factors (lipids, blood pressure, etc.)
- Improved response to pharmacologic therapy, with the potential of reducing the dosage or the need for insulin or oral antidiabetic agents
- Improved energy level, muscular strength, flexibility, quality of life, and sense of well-being.

Precautions and Considerations

Because many people with diabetes have not been active and are deconditioned, exercise should be started cautiously at a low level and gradually increased to avoid adverse effects such as injury, hypoglycemia, or cardiac problems. Most adults with diabetes should have a physical examination, including a stress test, before beginning to exercise to rule out significant cardiovascular disease or silent ischemia and determine the presence of any diabetic complications. Strenuous activity is not recommended for patients with poor metabolic control and those with significant complications.

Patients being treated with insulin secretagogues, or insulin alone or in combination are susceptible to hypoglycemia during or as much as 12 hours after exercising. To prevent hypoglycemia, these patients should use self-monitoring of blood glucose (SMBG) both before and after exercising to determine their response to varying degrees of physical activity. Appropriate consumption of snacks and modification of pharmacotherapy, as needed, can help avoid most problems. More importantly, establishing and following a regular exercise program can reduce the likelihood of exercise-induced episodes of hypoglycemia.

Exercise Prescription

Any exercise prescription should be individualized to account for patient interests, physical status and capacity, and motivation. Although having a planned program of physical activity is ideal, exercise is so important and beneficial that just getting patients moving is a worthwhile initial goal. Patients should choose activities that are appropriate for their general physical condition and lifestyle, start slowly, and work up to the goal of performing an aerobic activity at 50% to 70% of maximum oxygen uptake at least three to four times per week, with a minimum duration of 20 minutes per session (ideally 30 to 40 minutes). Weight reduction is enhanced by exercising five to six times per week. Recommended aerobic activities include:
- Walking at a moderate pace (3 to 5 miles/hour)
- Biking and stationary cycling
- Lap swimming and aerobic water exercises.

Muscle-strengthening exercises such as lifting light weights also should be included in an exercise program, as well as flexibility stretches during warm-ups and cool-downs.

Guidelines for safe exercise should be reviewed with patients (Table 6.1). Recommendations for a practical exercise prescription are outlined in Table 6.2.

TABLE 6.1 — GENERAL EXERCISE GUIDELINES

- Exercise stress test should be performed in most adults with diabetes to rule out significant cardiovascular disease or silent ischemia.
- Start slowly at a low level; gradually increase intensity and frequency.
- Carry identification including diabetes medical identification.
- Monitor blood glucose preexercise and postexercise.
- Be alert for signs of hypoglycemia during and several hours after exercising; carry appropriate readily available carbohydrate source.
- Closely monitor blood glucose when exercise intensity is increased.
- Drink sufficient fluids before, during, and after exercise to maintain adequate hydration.

6

TABLE 6.2 — PRACTICAL EXERCISE PRESCRIPTION

- Most individuals with type 2 diabetes are overweight and in poor cardiovascular health prior to initiating an exercise program. Exercise should be part of an overall beneficial change in lifestyle (diet modification, reduced stress, etc).
- Exercise programs can be of low, moderate, or high intensity. The exercise prescription needs to be individualized and account for the presence of macrovascular and microvascular complications, weighing the benefits vs risks in a given patient. Most individuals with type 2 diabetes should focus on a low-to-moderate intensity program that is easy to initiate and maintain.
- Low-to-moderate intensity exercise generally increases the heart rate up to approximately 60% of maximal heart rate. The maximal heart rate for an individual can be estimated by subtracting the age from 220 (maximal heart rate = 220 – age). Thus a 50-year-old individual exercising at a low-to-moderate intensity should keep the heart rate (220-50 = 170 x 60%) of no more than 100 beats per minute. Patients should be shown how to monitor their heart rate intermittently during exercise by palpation of the radial or brachial artery.

SUGGESTED READING

American Diabetes Association. Clinical practice recommendations 2002. Diabetes mellitus and exercise. *Diabetes Care*. 2002;25(suppl 1):S64-S68.

American Diabetes Association. *Medical Management of Non–insulin-dependent (Type II) Diabetes,* 3rd ed. Alexandria, Va: American Diabetes Association; 1994:22-39.

7 Oral Agents

The majority of patients with type 2 diabetes have less than ideal metabolic control despite our greater understanding of the underlying pathophysiologic mechanisms of hyperglycemia and the availability of a wide variety of new treatment options. Failure to achieve glycemic goals is related in part to a misconception by patients and caregivers that type 2 diabetes is a mild disease, and not as serious as type 1 diabetes. In fact, type 2 diabetes in many respects may have more severe consequences than type 1 diabetes because of the multiple cardiovascular risk factors and accelerated atherosclerosis associated with this form of diabetes.

Insulin resistance is an early and major cause of hyperglycemia and other metabolic abnormalities in type 2 diabetics (see Chapter 2, *Pathophysiology and Natural History*). Hyperglycemia in type 2 diabetes often coexists with several other metabolic abnormalities such as obesity, hypertension, dyslipidemia, and a procoagulant state, which themselves require prompt and aggressive diagnosis and treatment. Moreover, prolonged hyperglycemia leads to a worsening of the insulin resistance and endogenous insulin secretory inability (glucose toxicity), thus contributing to the primary and secondary oral agent failure rate. Aggressive management to reduce the hyperglycemia, which in some cases may require temporary insulin therapy, is necessary to reverse the glucose toxic state.

Pharmacologic therapy with oral antidiabetic agents is required when dietary modification and exercise therapy do not result in normalization or near normalization of metabolic abnormalities. Pharmacologic therapy should always be considered as adjunctive therapy to diet and exercise, and not as a substitute. Although maintaining an optimal diet and exercise regimen is difficult, it is important to emphasize that no pharmacologic therapy can be expected to be successful if the patient is not following some type of dietary and exercise program. Effort should be made to diagnose type 2 diabetes early in the natural history of the disease when nonpharmacologic therapy tends to be most effective.

Pathophysiologic Basis of Pharmacologic Therapy

The treatment strategies selected for managing type 2 diabetes are based on understanding the pathophysiology of hyperglycemia and the unique clinical expression of the associated metabolic abnormalities in an individual. Type 2 diabetes is characterized by three basic abnormalities that contribute to the development of hyperglycemia:

- Peripheral insulin resistance mainly in the skeletal muscle but also in the liver and adipose tissue
- Excessive glucose production by the liver
- Impaired insulin secretion by the pancreas.

Fasting and postprandial hyperglycemia vary considerably among individuals depending upon the extent, severity, and unique expression of each of these metabolic abnormalities, and these differences also play a role in the various responses to the different classes of oral antidiabetic agents. Such differences are exemplified by the lean and obese varieties of type 2 diabetes, which exhibit the same underlying pathophysiology but differ in the extent to which each abnormality contributes to the development of the hyperglycemic state. In lean type 2 diabetic patients, impaired insulin secretion is usually the predominant defect, while insulin resistance tends to be less severe than in the obese variety. Insulin resistance and hyperinsulinemia are the classic abnormalities of obese individuals with type 2 diabetes. In obese type 2 diabetics, the oral antidiabetic agents that do not stimulate insulin secretion tend to be as effective but safer than insulin secretagogues in terms of hypoglycemia when used early in the course of diabetes and insulin deficiency is not the predominant abnormality.

Importance of Controlling Postprandial Hyperglycemia

The evaluation of glycemic control and the response to antidiabetic therapy in type 2 diabetes has traditionally emphasized monitoring of fasting and preprandial glucose values. However, patients frequently demonstrate normal or near-normal preprandial glucose levels yet have distinctly abnormal postprandial glucose values. Postprandial hyperglycemia is often the first clinical abnormality present in those individuals who eventually go on to develop type 2 diabetes. Although it is not well recognized, postprandial hyperglycemia contributes significantly to elevated glycosylated hemoglobin (HbA$_{1C}$) and has been implicated in development of cardiovascular and other diabetic complications. Abnormal postprandial glucose values in pregnant diabetic women have also been shown to contribute to perinatal morbidity and mortality, and are more significantly correlated with adverse outcomes than fasting glucose levels. Many factors contribute to peak postprandial plasma glucose (eg, insulin resistance, impaired insulin secretion) but up to one third of the variance may be explained by differences in gastric emptying. Many type 2 diabetic patients demonstrate abnormally rapid gastric emptying after a high carbohydrate meal which may contribute to excessive postprandial glucose excursions.

The importance of controlling postprandial glucose needs to be recognized and treated with modification of diet and use of antidiabetic medication as required. Postprandial glucose levels are best evaluated 1 to 2 hours after meals by patients using home glucose monitoring devices. Action is suggested when the postprandial glucose value consistently exceeds 160 mg/dL with a goal of less than 140 mg/dL (Table 7.1). Recently, the American Association of Clinical Endocrinology (AACE) has published similar stringent guidelines for control of postprandial glucose with a 2-hour postprandial glucose goal of <140 mg/dL.

Intensive Therapy in Type 2 Diabetes

Several long-term studies of intensive diabetes management in both type 1 and type 2 diabetes have provided clear-cut evidence that near-normalization of glycemia can prevent and delay the development and progression of retinopathy, nephropathy, and neuropathy in the disease. Patients with type 2 diabetes obtain benefits from improved glycemic control because the severity and duration of hyperglycemia has a critical role in the development and progression of microvascular complications, regardless of the etiology of the hyperglycemia. Recent studies demonstrate not only a reduction in microvascular disease in type 2 diabetes with improved glycemic control, but also reductions in dyslipidemia and coronary artery disease.

The United Kingdom Prospective Diabetes Study (UKPDS) demonstrated the benefits of glucose control in over 5,000 individuals with newly diagnosed type 2 diabetes. The subjects were randomized into a conventional treatment group (nonpharmacologic diet treatment) with the goal to keep the fasting blood glu-

TABLE 7.1 — SUGGESTED GLYCEMIC GUIDELINES*		
Biochemical Index	**Goal**	**Action Suggested**
Fasting/prepran-dial glucose[†]	<80-120 mg/dL (4.4-6.7 mM)	<80 or >140 mg/dL (<4.4 or >7.8 mM)
Bedtime glucose[†]	100-140 mg/dL (5.6-7.8 mM)	<100 or >160 mg/dL (<5.6 or >8.9 mM)
Postprandial glucose[†]	<140 mg/dL (8.9 mM)	>160 mg/dL (10.0 mM)
Glycated hemo-globin[‡]	<7%	>8%

* Guidelines advocated by authors.
† Based on capillary blood glucose.
‡ Referenced to a nondiabetic range of 4% to 6% (mean 5%, SD 0.5%).

cose values less than 270 mg/dL and an intensive treatment group (sulfonylureas, insulin, or metformin) with the goal to keep the fasting blood glucose values less than 108 mg/dL. The average study duration of subjects was 11 years. Although the UKPDS was not ideally designed or conducted to achieve optimal glycemic control, several important messages have been derived from this study.

Most importantly, this study demonstrated a highly statistically significant reduction in microvascular disease in the intensive treatment group on the same order of magnitude as occurred in the Diabetes Control and Complications Trial (DCCT) in type 1 diabetes (Table 7.2). In the UKPDS, the difference in HbA_{1C} between the conventional and intensive treatment groups was only 0.9% compared with a 2% difference observed in the DCCT.

Improved glucose control led to a borderline statistically significant reduction in myocardial in-

TABLE 7.2 — UNITED KINGDOM PROSPECTIVE DIABETES STUDY: INTENSIVE BLOOD-GLUCOSE CONTROL		
	Change in Risk (%)	**P Value**
Any diabetes-related end point	↓ 12	0.025
Myocardial infarctions	↓ 16	0.052
Microvascular disease	↓ 25	0.0099

Adapted from: United Kingdom Prospective Diabetes Study (UKPDS) Group. *Lancet.* 1998;352:837-853.

farctions, although to a lesser extent than the reduction seen with the microvascular complications. Several large long-term studies are currently ongoing that directly assess the effect of glucose control on cardiovascular event risk reduction.

The natural history of type 2 diabetes was clearly demonstrated in both treatment groups, namely that there was a definite secondary failure rate (~7% per year) in all subjects (Figure 7.1). Part of the explanation for the high secondary failure rate may be that subjects were diagnosed relatively late in the natural history of the disease, as they are in the United States; on average, more than 5 years after onset of hyperglycemia. In this situation, the disease process would be well established and therapeutic interventions less effective to prevent the natural progression of the disease. Another likely possibility is that the mechanism of action of the therapeutic agents utilized did not significantly impact one or more of the major pathophysiologic abnormalities of type 2 diabetes such as insulin resistance and β-cell dysfunction.

To date there are no published reports demonstrating any serious adverse effects of near normalization of the glucose values in type 2 diabetes other than

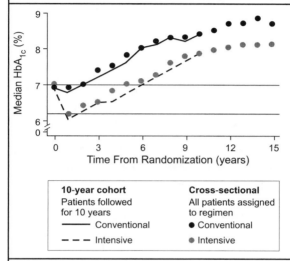

FIGURE 7.1 — UNITED KINGDOM PROSPECTIVE DIABETES STUDY CROSS-SECTIONAL AND 10-YEAR COHORT DATA FOR HbA$_{1c}$: INTENSIVE OR CONVENTIONAL TREATMENT

10-year cohort
Patients followed
for 10 years
—— Conventional
– – – Intensive

Cross-sectional
All patients assigned
to regimen
● Conventional
● Intensive

The trend toward loss of glycemic control was extended over the 10-year follow-up in the group of patients who received conventional treatment. HbA$_{1c}$ increased steadily over the 10 years. This can be seen in both the cross-sectional and 10-year cohort data. In patients who received intensive therapy, an initial decline in HbA$_{1c}$ was not sustained throughout the study. This result is similar to that seen in the conventional treatment group, confirming that type 2 diabetes worsens over time. A comparable result was seen over the course of the study with regard to fasting plasma glucose (FPG) levels—a gradual increase among patients who received conventional treatment and an initial reduction followed by deterioration among patients who received intensive treatment.

Adapted from: United Kingdom Prospective Diabetes Study (UKPDS) Group. *Lancet.* 1998;352:837-853.

weight gain and hypoglycemia. Thus, similar intensive management strategies, including all facets of diabetes care, that are applied rigorously to achieve normal or near-normal glycemia are warranted for patients with type 2 diabetes and should be attempted whenever possible.

The American Diabetes Association has responded to the implications of these studies by revising its therapeutic glycemic goals to advocate tighter metabolic control in both type 1 and type 2 diabetes (Table 7.1). Intensive therapy with diet, exercise, and antidiabetic agents alone or in combination (including insulin) is the most effective way to achieve these goals in patients with type 2 diabetes.

Diabetes Prevention Study Results

There have been several studies recently completed that have demonstrated that type 2 diabetes can be prevented or delayed. These studies have used several different interventions, including oral antidiabetic agents and intensive lifestyle modifications, in study subjects with impaired glucose tolerance (normal fasting glucose and a 2-hour value between 140 and 199 mg/dL following a 75-g glucose load).

■ Diabetes Prevention Program

The Diabetes Prevention Program (DPP) is an NIH-funded long-term study that was designed to determine whether diabetes could be prevented or delayed in people who had risk factors for developing type 2 diabetes. The risk factors for type 2 diabetes include:

- A family of history of type 2 diabetes
- Being overweight
- High blood pressure or abnormal cholesterol levels

- Gestational diabetes and/or a baby over 9 lbs
- A member of an ethnic group who has a high incidence of diabetes (Native American Indians, Latinos, Pacific Islanders, Asian Indians, and African Americans).

The participants of this study had glucose levels that were above the normal range but not quite in the diabetic range (impaired glucose tolerance or IGT). The participants were put into one of four treatment groups. The first group was the intensive lifestyle group; they exercised at least 150 minutes a week and lost 10 to 15 pounds over the $3\frac{1}{2}$ year duration of the study. The other three groups were put on metformin (Glucophage), troglitazone (Rezulin), or placebo, with only minimal lifestyle changes.

The DPP ended 1 year early because of the remarkable results gathered from 25 research institutions around the United States that including more than 4,000 subjects. Compared with placebo group, the subjects randomized to the intensive lifestyle group reduced their chances of developing type 2 diabetes by an impressive 58%. The individuals who were given metformin with minimal lifestyle changes showed a reduction in the development of diabetes by 31% over the 3-year study, compared with the placebo group. There was also a significant reduction in the conversion to type 2 diabetes in the troglitazone group, although this group was only on medication for an average of 10 months of the study because it was withdrawn from the study due to liver toxicity. The DPP is only one of several prevention trials recently completed demonstrating that intensive lifestyle can reduce the incidence of type 2 diabetes in individuals who are at high risk.

■ Troglitazone in the Prevention of Diabetes Study

The Troglitazone in the Prevention of Diabetes (TRIPOD) study is a second prevention trial that demonstrated several important findings. The first important result was that diabetes could be prevented and delayed with troglitazone (400 mg/day) by 56% compared with the placebo group in a cohort of high-risk nonpregnant, nondiabetic Hispanic women who had a recent history of gestational diabetes. In addition, metabolic studies performed during and after the study demonstrated prolonged pancreatic or β-cell preservation of function in the troglitazone-treated group even after the drug was discontinued. Although troglitazone is no longer on the market, this study suggests that similar benefits may be achieved with the other insulin sensitizers that are available (rosigliltazone [Avandia] and pioglitazone [Actos]).

■ Stop Non–Insulin-Dependent Diabetes Mellitus Study

The results of the 3-year Stop Non–insulin-dependent Diabetes Mellitus (NIDDM) study was also recently released demonstrating that a carbohydrate absorption inhibitor (acarbose) reduced or prevented the development of type 2 diabetes in an IGT group of subjects by approximately 23%.

The onset of diabetes can be delayed or prevented by several interventions including intensive lifestyle modification, metformin, a glitazone, and acarbose. There are several other prevention trials underway that will give us further insight on how to reduce the morbidity and mortality of diabetes. These studies have demonstrated the benefits of diagnosing individuals who will eventually go on to develop type 2 diabetes and treating them as early as possible in their natural history of the disease.

Oral Antidiabetic Agents

Oral medication should be initiated when 3 months of diet and exercise alone are unable to achieve or maintain plasma glucose levels within these glycemic guidelines. If patients are symptomatic, oral antidiabetic agents or insulin should be initiated immediately in concert with diet and exercise. Current therapy for the treatment of hyperglycemia of type 2 diabetes includes the following oral antidiabetic agents:

- The thiazolidinediones rosiglitazone and pioglitazone
- The biguanide metformin
- The alpha-glucosidase inhibitors acarbose and miglitol
- First- and second-generation sulfonylureas
- The D-phenylalanine derivative nateglinide
- The meglitinide repaglinide.

Until recently (before the availability of the nonsulfonylurea antidiabetic agents in the United States), approximately 35% of type 2 patients were treated with insulin. The number has been gradually decreasing with the advent of newer oral agents. In the United States, approximately two thirds of adults with type 2 diabetes use oral therapy during the first 5 years after diagnosis; this figure drops to about one third after a 20-year duration of diabetes. One of the explanations for this secondary failure rate of oral agents is that as the disease duration progresses, the endogenous insulin secretory ability of the pancreas diminishes, and the need for exogenous insulin increases. It is possible that by intensifying glycemic control early and by using non-insulin secreting oral agents and "resting" the pancreas, one can possibly delay this consistently observed β-cell exhaustion phenomenon.

Oral antidiabetic agents have different pharmacokinetics, potency, metabolism, and mechanisms of action that influence the choice of medication to use for initial and combination therapy (Table 7.3). Careful examination of the patient's metabolic profile, including weight, cholesterol levels, presence of glucose toxicity, duration of diabetes, and concomitant use with other oral agents, will dictate the best oral agent to use initially and in combination to achieve glycemic control. In general, oral agents are contraindicated in patients who:

- Are pregnant or lactating
- Are seriously ill
- Have significant kidney or liver disease
- Have demonstrated allergic reactions.

In addition, patients with significant and prolonged hyperglycemia with marked symptoms such as polyuria, polydipsia, or weight loss should be considered for temporary insulin therapy before considering the institution of oral agents. The rationale for insulin therapy is to acutely treat hyperglycemia to reduce glucotoxicity and enable the oral agents to be more effective.

Thiazolidinediones

The thiazolidinediones (or glitazones) are one of the newest classes of antidiabetic agents to be approved in the United States for the therapy of type 2 diabetes. These compounds work mainly to reduce insulin resistance in skeletal muscle, adipose tissue, and liver. At least some of their action involves stimulation of nuclear receptors called peroxisome proliferator-activated receptors (PPARs) that regulate gene transcription of a number of proteins involved in glucose and lipid metabolism. There are three types of PPAR receptors: PPARα, PPARβ, and PPARγ. Most of the initial interest in these receptors was generated by the knowledge that the thiazolidinediones are synthetic activators of PPARγ and this activation is associated with reducing insulin resistance. The exact mechanism by which activation of PPARγ improves insulin action is unknown but involves modifications in the expression of specific gene products and activity of pivotal enzymes of insulin signaling. PPARγ is highly expressed in adipose tissue but is also found in other tissues including skeletal muscle, liver, pancreas, macrophages, monocytes, and other cells of the vasculature.

Since insulin resistance is one of the earliest and major defects of type 2 diabetes and may predate the development of hyperglycemia by many years, these agents have the potential to have a large impact on the natural history of type 2 diabetes if used early in the course of the disease. The thiazolidinediones also have a major role in achieving and maintaining glucose control when used alone and in combination with other oral agents and insulin. Their efficacy to decease plasma glucose is well established with reductions in HbA_{1C} of 1% to 2%.

One of the most significant recent observations has been the ability of the glitazones to reduce cardiovascular risk factors including markers of vascular inflammation. This information is particularly important considering that cardiovascular disease is the major cause of morbidity and mortality in type 2 diabetes. Thus, these agents may not only delay or prevent the development of type 2 diabetes, but possibly influence development of premature cardiovascular disease as well.

■ Troglitazone

Troglitazone, which was the first thiazolidinedione marketed in the United States, was withdrawn from clinical use in March 2000 because of idiosyncratic hepatotoxicity with rare cases of liver failure,

TABLE 7.3 — CHARACTERISTICS OF CURRENTLY AVAILABLE ORAL ANTIDIABETIC AGENTS				
Generic Name	Trade Name	Recommended Starting Dose (mg)	Recommended Maximum Dose (mg)	Duration of Action (h)
SULFONYLUREAS*				
First Generation				
Acetohexamide	Dymelor	125 bid	750 bid	10-14
Chlorpropamide	Diabinese	250 qd	500 qd	60
Tolazamide	Tolinase	100 qd	500 bid	12-24
Tolbutamide	Orinase	250 bid	1000 tid	6-12
Second Generation				
Glimepiride	Amaryl	1-2 qd	8 qd	24
Glipizide	Glucotrol	5 qd	20 bid	12-24
Glipizide (extended release)	Glucotrol XL	5 qd	20 qd	24
Glyburide	DiaBeta, Micronase	2.5-5 qd	10 bid	16-24
	Glynase PresTab	1.5-3 qd	6 bid	12-24

GLINIDES				
Meglitinide†				
Repaglinide	Prandin	0.5 bid-qid w/meals	4 qid w/meals	2-4
D-Phenylalanine Derivative‡				
Nateglinide	Starlix	120 tid w/meals	120 tid w/meals	2-4
THIAZOLIDINEDIONES†				
Pioglitazone	Actos	15-30 qd	45 qd	24
Rosiglitazone	Avandia	4 qd	8 qd or 4 bid	24
BIGUANIDE§				
Metformin	Glucophage	500 with dinner	2550	Plasma elimination half-life ≈6.2 h
	Glucophage XR	500 qd	2000	Plasma elimination half-life ≈24 h
BIGUANIDE/SULFONYLUREA				
Glyburide/metformin	Glucovance	1.25/250 qd w/meals	2.5/500 qd w/meals	Plasma elimination half-life ≈ 10 h

Continued

Generic Name	Trade Name	Recommended Starting Dose (mg)	Recommended Maximum Dose (mg)	Duration of Action (h)
ALPHA-GLUCOSIDASE INHIBITORS[§]				
Acarbose	Precose	25 tid w/meals	100 tid w/meals	Not absorbed systemically
Miglitol	Glyset	25 tid w/meals	50 tid w/meals	

* Starting dosage for elderly and lean adults with diabetes may need to be reduced by up to 50%.

† Selection of initial dose depends on the patient's glucose level.

‡ Starting dosage may be reduced by 50% when patients are near the HbA$_{1C}$ goal.

§ The dosage of metformin, acarbose, and miglitol must be titrated slowly to limit gastrointestinal side effects.

Modified from: *Physicians' Desk Reference*, 56th ed. Montvale, NJ: Medical Economics Data Production Company; 2002.

leading to transplantation or death. After considerable clinical experience to date, rosiglitazone or pioglitazone do not appear to be associated with such fulminant idiosyncratic hepatotoxicity.

■ Rosiglitazone

Rosiglitazone is a thiazolidinedione that reduces peripheral insulin resistance in multiple tissues (muscle, adipose, and liver). It differs from troglitazone, having a shorter half-life (4 hour vs 16-34 hour), no enterohepatic recirculation, minimal induction of the hepatic cytochrome P450 enzyme CYP 34A, and primary urinary excretion (vs feces for troglitazone). It is currently indicated for use as monotherapy and in combination with sulfonylureas or metformin.

In the initial US placebo-controlled clinical trials of over 2,526 subjects previously treated with diet alone or antidiabetic medication(s), rosiglitazone monotherapy was shown to reduce the fasting plasma glucose values by up to an average of 58 mg/dL (4 mg/day) and 76 mg/dL (8 mg/day) compared with the placebo arm in a 26-week monotherapy study. In addition, with monotherapy the glycosylated hemoglobin was reduced by up to 1.5% in the 8 mg/day dosage group compared with placebo. Rosiglitazone may be given once daily or two divided doses. It is slightly more effective when given twice daily. When compared directly with maximum stable doses of glyburide, rosiglitazone reduced fasting plasma glucose by 25 mg/dL (4 mg/day) and 41 mg/dL (8 mg/day) compared with 30 mg/dL glucose reduction with glyburide (up to 15 mg/day). Although the reduction in HbA_{1C} was similar, the glycemic benefits were more sustained for rosiglitazone after 52 weeks. Importantly, with rosiglitazone, C-peptide, insulin, and proinsulin levels were significantly reduced, whereas they were increased in the glyburide-treated patients. Compared with glyburide or placebo, rosiglitazone has also been

7

shown to improve the proinsulin-to-insulin ratio in a dose-dependent manner. Such information is consistent with an insulin-sparing effect of rosiglitazone on the pancreas.

The addition of rosiglitazone for patients inadequately controlled on a sulfonylurea has proven to be an effective combination. In clinical trials of more than 1216 patients with type 2 diabetes, rosiglitazone at a dose of 2 mg bid or 4 qd was added to a sulfonylurea. At these doses, the mean reduction in fasting glucose from baseline values ranged from –25 to –38 mg/dL and in HbA_{1C} from –0.3% to –0.9%. When adding rosiglitazone, the dose of sulfonylurea should remain unchanged unless hypoglycemia occurs, then the dose of the sulfonylurea should be decreased.

Rosiglitazone has been shown to be effective when added to patients failing maximum metformin therapy. In a large, double-blind, placebo-controlled trial, 348 patients with type 2 diabetes failing maximal metformin therapy (2.5 g/day) were randomized to the addition of placebo, or 4 mg/day or 8 mg/day of rosiglitazone. After 26 weeks, fasting plasma glucose was reduced by 40 mg/dL in the 4-mg rosiglitazone/metformin group and by 53 mg/dL in the 8-mg rosiglitazone/metformin group (Figure 7.2). The time course of these effects is shown in Figure 7.3. Mean HbA_{1C} was reduced by 1.0% with the 4-mg dose and 1.2% with the 8-mg dose. Of those patients receiving maximum metformin and 8-mg rosiglitazone, 28% achieved an HbA_{1C} of <7%. Additionally, β-cell function measured by the homeostasis model assessment (HOMA) improved significantly with addition of rosiglitazone in a dose-dependent manner.

As with sulfonylureas, the current dose of metformin should be continued when adding rosiglitazone to the treatment regimen. Although unlikely, the dose of metformin should be reduced if hypoglycemia occurs with combination therapy.

86

FIGURE 7.2 — CHANGE IN FASTING PLASMA GLUCOSE CONCENTRATIONS AT WEEK 26 IN PATIENTS TAKING METFORMIN AND ROSIGLITAZONE COMPARED WITH TAKING METFORMIN ALONE

Comparison With Baseline

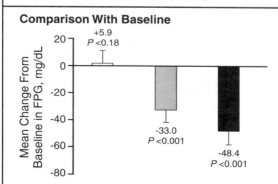

Comparison With Control Group at 26 Weeks

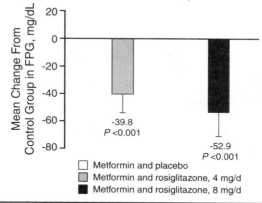

☐ Metformin and placebo
▨ Metformin and rosiglitazone, 4 mg/d
■ Metformin and rosiglitazone, 8 mg/d

Abbreviation: FPG, fasting plasma glucose.

To convert from milligrams per deciliter to millimoles per liter, multiply by 0.0555. Error bars indicate 95% confidence interval.

Fonseca V, et al. *JAMA*. 2000;283:1699.

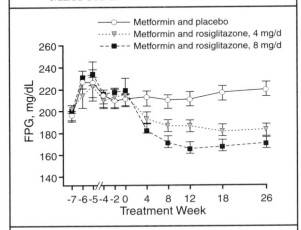

FIGURE 7.3 — MEAN FASTING PLASMA GLUCOSE CONCENTRATIONS OVER TIME IN PATIENTS TAKING METFORMIN ALONE COMPARED WITH PATIENTS TAKING METFORMIN AND ROSIGLITAZONE

Abbreviation: FPG, fasting plasma glucose.

To convert from milligrams per deciliter to millimoles per liter, multiply by 0.0555. Error bars indicate standard error.

Fonseca V, et al. *JAMA*. 2000;283:1699.

Rosiglitazone monotherapy can be associated with small increases in LDL cholesterol as well as large increases in HDL cholesterol (up to 19%). There is no change in the total cholesterol (TC)-to-HDL or LDL-to-HDL cholesterol ratio. In a recent study of rosiglitazone 8 mg/day for 24 weeks, LDL cholesterol increased 8% during the first 8 weeks and was stable subsequently. The increase in LDL cholesterol was paralleled by improvement in LDL density (to less dense, more buoyant particles). Seventy-one percent of the diabetic patients with small dense and potentially more atherogenic LDL had an increase in the

LDL density with rosiglitazone. Thus, some of the increase in LDL levels following rosiglitazone therapy is due to an increase in the size rather than the number of LDL particles. In this study, HDL 2 increased by 17% by week 8 with minimal change in HDL 3. Such effects in LDL and HDL are potentially antiatherogenic. Several studies have now shown an increase in the LDL-to-apolipoprotein B ratio consistent with a change in the composition of LDL particles from small, dense to a larger, more buoyant, potentially less atherogenic particles. Generally, despite significant decreases in FFA levels of more than 20% with rosiglitazone, the long-term effects on triglycerides are neutral. However, when rosiglitazone was combined with an HMG-CoA reductase inhibitor, reductions in LDL-cholesterol of 40% and triglycerides of 28% were reported.

Recent evidence indicates that rosiglitazone may have benefits in addition to those on glucose and lipids. There is now evidence of improvements in β-cell function, fibrinolytic activity, and reduced blood pressure following rosiglitazone therapy. Rosiglitazone at 8 mg/day for 1 year has been associated with reductions in systolic blood pressure of 3.5 mm Hg and diastolic blood pressure of 2.7 mm Hg. Rosiglitazone has been shown to reduce urinary albumin excretion, lower both plasminogen activator inhibitor-1 antigen and activity levels, and tissue plasminogen activator. Rosiglitazone has also recently been shown to exert widespread antiinflammatory effects in the vasculature as well as improved arterial reactivity. These changes have the potential for beneficial effects on diabetic vascular disease and development of cardiovascular events. Several long-term studies are currently underway with rosiglitazone that address diabetes prevention, progression of β-cell function, and cardiovascular outcomes.

Although the combination of rosiglitazone with exogenous insulin is not approved for clinical use, 8 mg daily of rosiglitazone added to insulin has been reported to reduce HbA$_{1C}$ by 1.2% despite a 12% mean reduction of insulin dosage.

Side Effects of Rosiglitazone

The incidence of ALT elevations of greater than three times the upper limit of normal for rosiglitazone was 0.2% compared with 0.2% for placebo in the initial clinical trials. When adjusted for duration of exposure, rosiglitazone had 0.35 cases of ALT elevation per 100 patient years, compared with 0.59 cases for placebo and 0.78 cases for active control (sulfonylureas or metformin). Liver monitoring guidelines are currently at baseline, every other month for the first year, and periodically thereafter.

On average, a 3% increase in body weight was observed after 6 to 12 months of therapy with rosiglitazone (2 to 3 kg). Weight gain was higher when rosiglitazone was given alone compared with when it was combined with metformin (0.7 to 2 kg).

Edema occurred in 4.8% of patients on rosiglitazone compared with 1.3% on placebo. In clinical trials, withdrawals due to edema were similar for placebo (0.2%) and rosiglitazone (0.2%).

Anemia was reported in 1.9% of rosiglitazone-treated patients compared with 0.7% of placebo-treated patients. Dose-dependent reductions in hemoglobin (up to approximately 1 g/dL) and hematocrit (3% to 5%) occur during the initial 8 weeks of therapy with rosiglitazone 8 mg/day, but stabilize thereafter.

Although these side effects are probably not clinically significant, close monitoring is recommended in patients with New York Heart Association class III and IV congestive heart failure. One year echocardiographic studies of rosiglitazone 8 mg/day demonstrate no adverse effects on cardiac structure or function but significant decreases in diastolic blood pressure. Two-year data has been analyzed and is consistent with the 1-year findings.

Prescribing Rosiglitazone

When prescribing rosiglitazone, the dosage should be low initially (4 mg qd) and then titrated up to 8 mg qd or 4 mg po bid for the maximum effect. In combination with a sulfonylurea, rosiglitazone is currently approved for doses up to 4 mg/day. Large, well-controlled clinical trials studying doses of greater than 4 mg/day are currently underway. The onset of action is evident at 2 weeks, but may require up to 12 weeks for maximal benefits to occur. Liver function tests should be monitored according to prescribing guidelines. Rosiglitazone does not need to be taken with food.

■ Pioglitazone

Pioglitazone, the newest thiazolidinedione, also reduces peripheral insulin resistance and hepatic glucose production. Pioglitazone is indicated for use as monotherapy or in combination with metformin, sulfonylureas, or insulin. Six registration studies (three monotherapy, three combination therapy) formed the basis of the FDA approval.

The monotherapy studies included 865 patients with type 2 diabetes. In general, there was a 1.4% to 1.6% reduction in HbA_{1C} observed with the highest dose of pioglitazone (45 mg/day) over a treatment period of 16 to 26 weeks. Interestingly, in treatment-naive patients with a short duration of diabetes, greater reductions of HbA_{1C} and FPG were observed.

In the combination therapy studies, pioglitazone or placebo was added to patients failing sulfonylureas, metformin, or insulin. There was a significant 0.8% to 1.3% reduction in the HbA_{1C} in these studies when the 30 mg/day dose of pioglitazone was used. Addition of 15 mg or 30 mg pioglitazone leads to dose-dependent reductions to patients on exogeneous insulin in both fasting plasma glucose and HbA$_{1C}$ levels (Figure 7.4). In addition, interim analysis of ongoing longer term studies with pioglitazone indicates prolonged efficacy in a similar fashion to what has been seen with troglitazone and rosiglitazone.

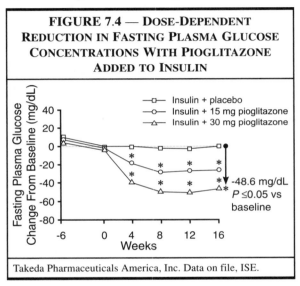

FIGURE 7.4 — DOSE-DEPENDENT REDUCTION IN FASTING PLASMA GLUCOSE CONCENTRATIONS WITH PIOGLITAZONE ADDED TO INSULIN

Takeda Pharmaceuticals America, Inc. Data on file, ISE.

Pioglitazone used as monotherapy and in combination resulted in a significant mean percent decrease in triglycerides (up to 15%) and significant mean percent increases in HDL (up to 19%) with no consistent effects on LDL or total cholesterol levels. As with all thiazolidinediones, treatment with pioglitazone has also been shown to shift fat distribution from visceral to subcutaneous areas.

Side Effects of Pioglitazone

In clinical studies worldwide, over 4500 subjects have received pioglitazone and there was no evidence of drug-induced hepatotoxicity or elevation of ALT levels. During placebo-controlled clinical trials in the United States, a total of four of 1526 patients (0.26%) treated with pioglitazone and two of 793 placebo-treated patients (0.25%) had ALT values ≥ three times the upper limit of normal. After long-term open label treatment with pioglitazone (up to 88 weeks), 11 of 2561 pioglitazone-treated patients (0.43%) reported ALT values ≥ three times the upper limit of normal. Upon follow-up testing, the ALT elevations in all patients were reversible. The frequency of postmarketing reports of abnormal liver tests is consistent with that suggested by clinical trials.

The main treatment-related side effect was peripheral edema. Incidence ranged from 4.8% as monotherapy to 15.3% in combination with insulin. Patients with New York Heart Association class III or IV heart failure were not studied. Weight increases were seen during treatment with pioglitazone, and as observed with rosiglitazone, most weight gain occurred in the early period of treatment and was correlated with improvements in glycemic control (HbA_{1c}). Across all clinical studies, mean hemoglobin values declined by 2% to 4% in patients treated with pioglitazone. These changes primarily occurred within the first 4 to 12 weeks of therapy and most likely are related to increased plasma volume.

Prescribing Information

Dosing of pioglitazone should be titrated up to a maximum effective daily dose of 45 mg as monotherapy only and up to 30 mg in combination therapy. Pioglitazone is always administered once daily and can be taken without regard to food. Onset of activity has been observed as early as 2 weeks with maximum effects seen in 8 weeks. Liver function testing should be consistent with current package insert (prior to the initiation of therapy, every other month for the first year, and then periodically).

■ Summary

When used in the appropriate clinical situation, the thiazolidinedione class of oral agents can have a significant impact on the metabolic management of type 2 diabetes. The novel mechanism of action of thiazolidinediones to improve insulin resistance has unique potential in new onset type 2 diabetes. Many of the greatest benefits of these agents may be in patients who are in the early stages of developing diabetes and premature cardiovascular disease.

Metformin

Metformin (Glucophage) is a biguanide that works by:
- Mainly suppressing excessive hepatic glucose production
- Increasing glucose utilization in peripheral tissues to a lesser degree.

Metformin may also improve glucose levels by reducing intestinal glucose absorption. Because metformin does not stimulate endogenous insulin secretion, hypoglycemia does not usually occur when this drug is used alone, although hypoglycemia may occur if metformin is taken with insulin, a sulfonylurea, or an excessive amount of alcohol. Metformin is not metabolized and is excreted unchanged by the kidneys. Metformin is often used as initial pharmacologic therapy in patients failing diet and exercise therapy.

Metformin is effective as monotherapy or in combination with sulfonylureas. The combinations of metformin with thiazolidinediones, alpha-glucosidase inhibitors, the glinides, or insulin has also been shown to be safe and effective. In short-term studies, metformin can be added to the regimens of patients who have not responded initially to sulfonylureas (primary treatment failure) or patients who responded initially to sulfonylureas, but who subsequently have deterioration of glycemic control (secondary treatment failure). Sulfonylureas can also be added to the regimens of patients failing metformin therapy. The combination of metformin and a sulfonylurea often achieves a better glycemic response than either agent given alone. When metformin is added to sulfonylureas, the dose of the sulfonylurea should be maintained.

Treatment with metformin has beneficial effects on plasma lipids that are greater than expected from improved glucose control alone (it lowers triglyceride and low-density lipoprotein [LDL] cholesterol levels while increasing high-density lipoprotein [HDL] cholesterol). In addition, metformin therapy has been associated with weight loss or less weight gain than other oral antidiabetic agents. This may be particularly helpful in obese patients with type 2 diabetes.

■ **Side Effects of Metformin**
The major side effects of metformin are:
- Gastrointestinal effects, consisting mainly of mild diarrhea or "loose stools"
- Anorexia
- Nausea
- Abdominal discomfort.

For most patients, these side effects:
- Are transient
- Are dose related
- Tend to decrease with chronic therapy.

They can be minimized by:
- Slow dosage titration
- Decreasing the dosage (sometimes only temporarily)
- Taking metformin with meals.

Lactic acidosis is a rare complication of metformin therapy but has a high mortality rate. Most of the cases of metformin-associated lactic acidosis occurred in patients for whom the drug was contraindicated, ie, patients with renal dysfunction. Metformin should not be prescribed if the serum creatinine is greater than 1.5 mg/dL in men or greater than 1.4 mg/dL in women. In patients over 80 years of age, it is recommended that a 24-hour urine collection be obtained to measure creatinine clearance, which is a better indicator of kidney function. Metformin is also contraindicated in patients with significant hepatic disease, cardiac insufficiency, alcohol abuse, and any hypoxic condition or history of lactic acidosis. Metformin should not be used in any patient with congestive heart failure (compensated or uncompensated) who is currently on a loop diuretic and/or digoxin. Metformin should be temporarily discontinued at the time of or prior to any dye studies so that serum metformin levels are low if the patient develops renal failure from the dye. Metformin should be withheld for 48 hours subsequent to dye studies and reinstated only after renal function has been evaluated and found to be normal. In any patient who is hospitalized with an acute severe illness, metformin should be temporarily discontinued until the condition improves. During such circumstances, insulin is generally the preferred form of therapy.

■ Prescribing Metformin

The manufacturer's recommended starting dose for metformin is 500 mg twice a day or 850 mg once a day given with meals. However, we suggest an initial dose of 500 mg/day with dinner for 1 week, then twice daily with breakfast and dinner to improve tolerability. The dosage should be titrated slowly, as needed, toward a maximum daily dose of 2550 mg. A third dose can be safely added at bedtime instead of at noon; compliance tends to be better. Metformin at bedtime works well to suppress hepatic glucose production overnight. Several weeks are required to observe the maximum effect of metformin once a stable dosage is achieved.

■ Metformin/Glyburide Combination

A new combination pill is available that consists of metformin and glyburide (1.25 mg glyburide combined with 250 mg metformin and 2.5 mg or 5.0 mg glyburide combined with 500 mg metformin) (Glucovance). In the monotherapy pivotal trials, Glucovance was more effective at lowering the HbA_{1C} and fasting and postprandial glucose values when compared with metformin or glyburide alone. Even though Glucovance combines two medications that have been available for many years, early combination therapy with two different drugs that have different mechanisms of action have shown advantages.

Glucophage also is available in an extended-release form (Glucophage XR). It can be taken once a day with equal efficacy compared with the short-acting form.

Alpha-Glucosidase Inhibitors

Acarbose (Precose) and miglitol (Glyset) are alpha-glucosidase inhibitors that slow the breakdown of complex carbohydrates (disaccharides and polysaccharides) into monosaccharides or glucose. The enzymatic generation and subsequent absorption of glucose is delayed and the postprandial blood glucose values, which are characteristically high in patients with type 2 diabetes, are reduced with these agents. The postprandial blood glucose level is often overlooked but can significantly contribute to prolonged hyperglycemia. Acarbose and miglitol are excellent pharmacologic agents to "spread the calories" which is recommended by the American Diabetes Association and have been shown to smooth out daytime glycemia.

■ Acarbose

Acarbose has proven to be an effective agent when used alone or in combination with other antidiabetic agents. Acarbose has been shown to reduce the mean postprandial glucose value by approximately 50 mg/dL and the fasting glucose by 10 to 20 mg/dL. Acarbose also lowers the postprandial integrated insulin levels, as less glucose is being presented to the pancreas at any one time. Acarbose does not stimulate insulin release and does not cause hypoglycemia when used alone. The average reduction in HbA_{1C} is usually 0.5% to 1.0%. The reduction in glycemia is related to the carbohydrate content of the diet. Generally, the greater the complex carbohydrate content of the diet, the larger the reduction in postprandial hyperglycemia. In addition, a recent large scale trial has demonstrated that when acarbose is given to patients with newly diagnosed diabetes (duration of up to 1 year) with poor metabolic control (baseline HbA_{1C} >10%), a 3.0% to 4.6% reduction in HbA_{1C} can be seen. Since acarbose primarily reduces the postprandial blood glucose and does not cause hypoglycemia, the drop in HbA_{1C} is usually not as dramatic as one would see with the sulfonylureas, which can cause hypoglycemia (the HbA_{1C} is an average of the highs and lows of plasma glucose).

The combined use of acarbose with metformin and/or insulin has been approved by the FDA. Acarbose has been used successfully with thiazolidinediones and repaglinide for the treatment of type 2 diabetes, although these latter two combinations are not yet approved by the FDA.

Side Effects of Acarbose

The main side effect of acarbose is flatulence. Soft stools or diarrhea and mild abdominal pain have also been reported. Many of the symptoms are dose related and transient, occurring with the highest frequency during the first 8 weeks of therapy. The symptoms are probably caused by the osmotic effect of undigested carbohydrates in the distal bowel. The most important factor in avoiding side effects is to titrate acarbose slowly. Because acarbose is not absorbed systemically to any significant degree and does not cause hypoglycemia, it has been suggested that it may be safer than some of the other oral agents in patients with kidney disease, in the elderly, and in children with type 2 diabetes.

Prescribing Acarbose

The recommended maintenance dosage of acarbose is 50 mg to 100 mg orally 3 times a day with meals. The suggested starting dosage of acarbose is 25 mg/day and should be titrated up slowly to the maintenance dosage of 50 mg to 100 mg tid to avoid side effects (Table 7.4).

■ Miglitol

Miglitol is a similar compound to acarbose that also has alpha-glucosidase inhibitor activity in the gut, thereby delaying or preventing the digestion and absorption of complex carbohydrates. In a similar fashion to acarbose, miglitol does not directly stimulate insulin secretion and does not cause hypoglycemia when used alone. The main clinical effect of miglitol is to lower the postprandial glucose value with additive effects of lowering postprandial insulin levels and a lesser reduction in the fasting plasma glucose values. The magnitude of reductions of the glycosylated hemoglobin values are on the same order of magni-

TABLE 7.4 — ACARBOSE/MIGLITOL DOSING INSTRUCTIONS FOR PATIENTS

1. You have been given acarbose/miglitol because your blood sugar control needs to be improved. Acarbose/miglitol is a very safe medication that has been proven effective in improving overall blood sugar control in people with diabetes.

2. Acarbose/miglitol works by delaying the absorption of glucose in the gut or delaying the digestion of carbohydrates and subsequent absorption of glucose.

3. Acarbose/miglitol reduces the rise in blood sugar that typically occurs after eating. Marked elevation in blood sugar after eating is a common yet important problem that often is overlooked.

4. Acarbose/miglitol *may* cause flatulence (excess gas), mild stomach pain, and/or diarrhea. These side effects tend to occur at the beginning of therapy and can be lessened by starting with a low dose of acarbose/miglitol and increasing the dose very slowly.

5. Suggested dosing schedule:
   Step 1: Start with 25 mg* at breakfast only for 1 week
   Step 2: Take 25 mg with breakfast and dinner for 1 week
   Step 3: Take 25 mg with breakfast, lunch, and dinner for 1 week
   Step 4: Take 50 mg with breakfast and 25 mg with lunch and dinner for 1 week
   Step 5: Take 50 mg with breakfast and dinner, and 25 mg with lunch for 1 week
   Step 6: Take 50 mg with breakfast, lunch, and dinner†

6. Do not go to a higher step if you are having bothersome gas, stomach pain, or diarrhea. Stay at the current step or go to a lower step until your symptoms improve.

7. It is extremely important to take acarbose/miglitol with the beginning of your meal. Acarbose/miglitol will be less effective at lowering your blood sugar if you take it more than 15 minutes before you eat.

---

* Break the 50-mg pill in half or use a pill cutter.
† Do not increase your dose further until you talk with your caregiver.

tude as seen with acarbose, although 50 mg tid of miglitol has been shown to be equivalent to 100 tid of acarbose in terms of efficacy. Miglitol can be safely added to all other oral agents on the market as well as with insulin.

Sides Effects of Miglitol

Flatulence is the main GI side effect experienced with miglitol therapy, however it may be better tolerated than other carbohydrate absorption inhibitors.

Prescribing Miglitol

The recommended maintenance dosage of miglitol is 25 mg to 50 mg orally three times a day with meals. The suggested starting dosage of miglitol is 25 mg/day and should be titrated up slowly to the maintenance dosage of 25 mg to 50 mg tid to avoid side effects (Table 7.4).

Sulfonylureas

Sulfonylureas work primarily by chronically stimulating pancreatic insulin secretion, which in turn reduces hepatic glucose output and increases peripheral glucose disposal.

Four first-generation sulfonylurea compounds have been available in the United States for the treatment of type 2 diabetes for over 20 years. They are:
- Acetohexamide
- Chlorpropamide
- Tolazamide
- Tolbutamide.

Two second-generation sulfonylurea compounds (glipizide and glyburide) were introduced in the United States in 1984 and another (glimepiride) more recently. Thus, the second-generation compounds are:

- Glimepiride
- Glipizide
- Glyburide.

The efficacy of the first- and second-generation sulfonylureas is similar, although second-generation agents are better formulated and have some advantages. Second-generation sulfonylureas:

- Are more potent on a per milligram basis
- Tend to produce fewer side effects
- Interact less frequently with other drugs.

Improved formulations of glipizide (Glucotrol XL) and glyburide (Glynase PresTab) are also available. In addition, the pharmacokinetics of some of these second-generation agents allow for more effective once-a-day dosing, which enhances compliance.

■ Side Effects of Sulfonylureas

Most of the side effects associated with sulfonylurea therapy are mild, infrequent, and occur less often with the second-generation agents; they include:

- Weight gain
- Hypoglycemia
- Mild gastrointestinal (GI) upset
- Skin reactions:
  - Rashes
  - Purpura
  - Pruritus.

Hyponatremia, fluid retention, and an Antabuse-like reaction to alcohol have also been reported with the use of chlorpropamide. The major complication of sulfonylurea therapy is severe hypoglycemia, which has been more of a problem with chlorpropamide than with any other agent because of its long half-life and duration of action. Hypoglycemia is also more common in individuals who consume large amounts of alcohol, skip meals, and in the elderly. Other reactions are rare and include hematologic reactions (leukopenia, thrombocytopenia, and hemolytic anemia) and cholestasis (with and without jaundice).

■ **Prescribing Sulfonylureas**

In general, therapy should be initiated at the lowest possible dose, especially in the elderly (Table 7.3). It is begun once daily, before breakfast, and increased progressively every 1 to 2 weeks until the desired therapeutic glycemic response is achieved or the maximum dose is reached. The dosing regimen is changed to twice daily when the daily dose approaches 50% or more of the maximum recommended dose. Dosing adjustments can also be made based on self-monitoring of blood glucose (SMBG) data. For example, if the patient's SMBG results show elevated fasting blood glucose values, then the evening dose should be titrated upward. If, on the other hand, the evening blood glucose values are elevated, then the morning dose can be raised.

Clinicians should focus on achieving satisfactory glycemic control based on glucose and HbA_{1c} levels and not concentrate solely on the patient's symptoms, which could lead to premature dosage discontinuation or dose reduction. In patients with glucose toxicity and markedly elevated glucose values (ie, >200-300 mg/dL), it may be necessary to use insulin temporarily to achieve glycemic control. Once glycemic control has been achieved for several days to weeks, the patient may be an appropriate candidate for oral agent therapy alone. Patients who do not achieve appropriate glycemic control in response to one or more oral agents should be promptly switched to or have insulin therapy added to the existing oral regimen.

In general, sulfonylureas should not be considered routinely as monotherapy for newly diagnosed obese patients with type 2 diabetes or in diabetic individuals failing nonpharmacologic therapy. Such patients usually have circulating hyperinsulinemia that can be further exacerbated if sulfonylureas are used. Sulfonylureas also lead to weight gain and can cause hypoglycemia. There is also some evidence to suggest that the early use of sulfonylureas may lead to premature β-cell exhaustion. In addition, concerns persist about the possible adverse effects of some sulfonylureas on cardiac function.

■ Second-Generation Sulfonylureas
Glimepiride

Glimepiride (Amaryl) is a relatively new sulfonylurea agent. Glimepiride therapy has been shown to improve overall glucose control without producing clinically meaningful increases in fasting insulin and C-peptide levels. It is the only sulfonylurea with a Food and Drug Administration (FDA)-approved indication for combination therapy with insulin. In recent studies, glimepiride has been shown to cause little or no weight gain or hypoglycemia.

The usual maintenance dosage is 1 mg to 4 mg once daily. The maximum recommended dosage is 8 mg once daily. After reaching a dose of 2 mg, further increases should be of no more than 2 mg at 1- to 2-week intervals based on the patient's blood glucose response.

Glipizide

Glipizide (Glucotrol, Glucotrol XL) is a second-generation sulfonylurea that is metabolized by the liver mainly to inactive products, reducing the risk of hypoglycemia. Glucotrol XL utilizes a controlled delivery system, and when compared with the immediate-release Glucotrol, the risk of hypoglycemia and the glucose and insulin responses to meals are similar although compliance is improved. Glipizide is particularly suited for the elderly or any patient with mild renal or liver dysfunction. Recommended dosing is normally 1 to 2 times daily for immediate-release glipizide. The long-acting extended-release formulation (Glucotrol XL) maintains therapeutic plasma levels effectively for 24 hours, and once-daily dosing is adequate in the majority of patients.

Glyburide

Glyburide (DiaBeta, Micronase, Glynase PresTab) is metabolized by the liver to mostly inert products that are excreted in the urine and bile. However, some of the by-products do have hypoglycemic activity and caution is advised, especially in patients with evidence of liver or kidney dysfunction. The duration of action is 16 to 24 hours, and recommended dosing is one to two times daily. A micronized particle formulation facilitates more rapid absorption (Glynase PresTab).

7

Glinides

■ **Meglitinide**
Repaglinide

An agent from the meglitinide class of compounds, repaglinide (Prandin), is available for monotherapy and in combination with metformin. It is unrelated to the sulfonylureas and is a benzoic acid derivative that closes ATP-sensitive potassium channels in pancreatic β-cells. This closure leads to depolarization and release of insulin in a glucose-dependent manner. Repaglinide causes a rapid rise and fall of insulin secretion when ingested 30 minutes or less prior to a meal and mimics the normal postprandial insulin response that follows ingestion of food. Repaglinide is generally not recommended in combination with sulfonylureas.

Although not FDA approved, repaglinide works well with carbohydrate absorption inhibitors such as acarbose and miglitol as well as the thiazolidinediones. A potentially useful triple combination oral antidiabetic regimen includes a thiazolidinedione in the morning, repaglinide with each meal, and metformin at bedtime. This triple combination addresses the three major physiological abnormalities observed in the pathogenesis of hyperglycemia in type 2 diabetes (insulin resistance, impaired insulin secretion, and excessive hepatic glucose production).

Prescribing Repaglinide

Repaglinide is taken before meals and the recommended dosage range is 0.5 mg to 4 mg preprandially, 2, 3, or 4 times a day according to the patient's meal pattern. Patients should be instructed that if they miss or add a meal they should omit or add the corresponding repaglinide dose. A maximum recommended daily dose is 16 mg.

Side Effects of Repaglinide

There is a small weight gain (3.3%) when treated with repaglinide as monotherapy and a low incidence of hypoglycemia. Since repaglinide is also cleared by the liver, it can be used in type 2 diabetic patients when renal impairment is present.

■ D-Phenylalanine Derivative
Nateglinide

This new agent from the D-phenylalanine class of compounds, nateglinide (Starlix) has recently been approved for type 2 diabetes as initial monotherapy and in combination with metformin. It is structurally distinct from all other available oral antidiabetic agents and exerts its glucose-lowering effect by rapid and transient effects on the ATP-sensitive potassium channels of pancreatic β-cells. Binding of nateglinide to the sulfonylurea receptor leads to membrane depolarization and influx of calcium into the β-cell. The increased intracellular calcium stimulates insulin release from secretory granules. Nateglinide, when taken orally up to 30 minutes prior to meals, is rapidly and almost completely absorbed. It stimulates pancreatic insulin secretion within 20 minutes, reaching peak insulin levels within 1 hour, returning to baseline levels within 4 hours of dosing. The extent of insulin secretion is glucose-dependent so that more insulin is secreted when needed and its effects are rapidly reversed when glucose levels decrease. Thus, insulin is secreted during the early phase after meals, reducing glucose spikes and minimizing prolonged insulin exposure and hypoglycemia.

Early insulin secretion released at the start of a meal suppresses hepatic glucose production and prevents exaggerated postprandial glucose levels. Early insulin secretion is impaired in patients with type 2 diabetes, leading to lack of suppression of hepatic glucose production and a rise in postprandial glucose levels. Nateglinide improves early insulin secretion through a fast-on, fast-off effect that mimics normal insulin secretion.

Postprandial or postmeal glucose excursions are a major component of HbA_{1C} and are frequently increased yet untreated. When HbA_{1C} is $\geq 7\%$, 90% of patients have a 2-hour plasma glucose above 200 mg/dL. Elevated 2-hour postprandial glucose levels are also associated with an increased incidence of cardiovascular disease in diabetic individuals. Although there are as yet no outcome studies for targeted postprandial glucose levels, the general consensus is that 2-hour postmeal glucose should be less than 140 to 160 mg/dL. These levels are now achievable with the new agents that target postprandial glucose control.

Studies have been conducted in both drug-naive type 2 diabetic patients as well as those previously treated with other antidiabetic agents. In drug-naive patients, 6 months treatment with nateglinide 120 mg three times daily before meals achieved comparable reductions in HbA_{1C} (1%) from placebo as 500 mg tid metformin with meals (1.1%). In both drug-naive and previously treated patients combined, nateglinide reduced HbA_{1C} 0.8% and metformin 1.2% from placebo. When nateglinide and metformin were combined for 6 months, the reduction in HbA_{1C} (1.9%) from placebo was greater than either agent given alone. The preferential effect of nateglinide on postprandial glucose levels compared with metformin was also evident in this study (Figure 7.5). Patients not achieving HbA_{1C} target levels also benefit from addition of nateglinide. Nateglinide 120 mg three times daily before meals added to metformin 1000 mg twice daily reduced HbA_{1C} an additional 0.6% compared with addition of a placebo.

Prescribing Nateglinide

Nateglinide is indicated as initial therapy, as an adjunct to diet and exercise, and in combination with metformin. Patients failing sulfonylureas do not achieve any additional benefit when nateglinide is switched or added. The recommended starting and maintenance dose of nateglinide, as monotherapy or in combination with metformin, is 120 mg prior to each main meal. Unlike other antidiabetic agents, dose titration is usually not required. If a meal is skipped, nateglinide should not be given. If patients are near the HbA_{1C} goal, a 60-mg dose of nateglinide may be sufficient when initiated as monotherapy or in combination with metformin. The dose also does not need to be adjusted in patients with mild to severe renal insufficiency or mild hepatic disease.

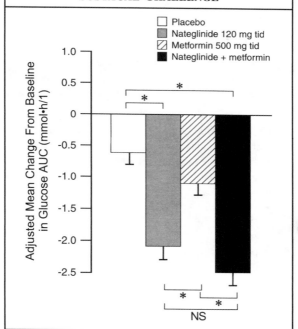

FIGURE 7.5 — COMPARISON OF NATEGLINIDE ON PPG LEVELS FOLLOWING SUSTACAL CHALLENGE

Abbreviations: AUC, area under the curve; PPG, postprandial glucose; NS, not significant; tid, three times/ day.

* $P \leq 0.0001$.

Adapted from: Horton ES, et al. *Diabetes Care*. 2000;23: 1663.

Side Effects of Nateglinide

Adverse events with nateglinide are similar to placebo. Small increases in mean uric acid levels (0.20-0.45 mg/dL) have been reported. During clinical trials, hypoglycemia was relatively uncommon (2.4% incidence vs placebo) and resulted in discontinuation of nateglinide in only 0.3% of patients. No severe hypoglycemia occurred requiring assistance of others. Minimal weight gain occurred with nateglinide, <1 kg from baseline values. Nateglinide is safe in elderly diabetic subjects and can be used in mild to severe renal insufficiency or mild hepatic insufficiency.

Monotherapy With Oral Antidiabetic Agents

The choice of therapy for type 2 diabetes has become more complicated as a result of the availability of several new classes of oral antidiabetic agents. Patients should be evaluated on an individual basis considering these variables:

- Age
- Weight
- Duration of diabetes
- Compliance
- Presence of dyslipidemia
- Duration and severity of hyperglycemia (glucose toxicity)
- Presence and degree of kidney, cardiac, and liver disease
- Presence of ulcer disease and other GI problems.

In general, the traditional approach to patients with type 2 diabetes failing nonpharmacologic therapy has been to start a sulfonylurea agent. However, this approach has been significantly altered by the additional availability of four new classes of antidiabetic medications. It is the authors' belief that sulfonylureas should no longer be used routinely as initial monotherapy for the obese patients with type 2 diabetes due to the more physiologic mechanisms of the new oral antihyperglycemic agents, and because of the real and potential adverse effects of sulfonylureas mentioned earlier. Therapeutic recommendations for several of
110

the commonly seen clinical presentations of patients with type 2 diabetes are described below.

■ Obese Patients With Newly Diagnosed Diabetes With/Without Dyslipidemia

Thiazolidinediones, metformin, or alpha-glucosidase inhibitors have the advantage of not inducing hypoglycemia or weight gain as monotherapy, which can occur with insulin secretagogues and insulin therapy. Either of these drugs is an appropriate choice after an unsuccessful 3-month trial of nonpharmacologic intervention. There is no risk of hypoglycemia because thiazolidinediones, metformin, and alpha-glucosidase inhibitors do not stimulate insulin secretion. Additional benefits of the thiazolidinediones and metformin include lowering of triglyceride levels and raising of HDL cholesterol. These effects are in addition to those resulting from improved glycemic control.

Sulfonylureas, in general, should be avoided in obese patients although they may be helpful if there is evidence of glucose toxicity (patients whose fasting blood glucose levels are consistently high, ie, >250 mg/dL) (see *Patients With Prolonged, Severe Hyperglycemia [Glucose Toxicity]*). Sulfonylureas in this situation are advantageous as they can be started at relatively high doses without the need for titrating because of the absence of GI side effects. At a later point in time and once glucose toxicity has subsided, a more physiologic oral agent could be tried and the sulfonylurea discontinued.

■ Thin Elderly Patients

Thin patients in general tend to be more insulin deficient and commonly require sulfonylureas or glinides as initial oral monotherapy. Caution should be used when prescribing any medication in the elderly, and starting doses need to be lower than those in younger patients. A thiazolidinedione or metformin may also be effective as monotherapy; however, caution should be used with metformin in the elderly who may have impaired renal function that is obscured by reduced muscle mass. Such individuals may have a serum creatinine level that is within the dosing guidelines (males <1.5 mg/dL; females <1.4 mg/dL), but may have reduced renal function. When unsure, creatinine clearance should be measured and metformin avoided when the creatinine clearance is less than 60 mL/min.

Thiazolidinediones or fast-acting insulin secretagogues can be used safely in patients with renal insufficiency. Sulfonylureas are usually effective, although the risk of hypoglycemia is higher in this population as they are more insulin sensitive because of their nonobese status. A glinide may be a good choice in such patients who eat inconsistently because of the rapid diminution of action and insulin levels that occur after ingestion of the drug. Alpha-glucosidase inhibitors also represent a safe approach because they are excreted independent of renal function, not absorbed systemically, and do not cause hypoglycemia.

■ Patients With Acceptable Fasting Glucose Values but Elevated Glycohemoglobin Levels

This scenario suggests the likelihood of elevated postprandial glucose levels, which can be confirmed by testing finger-stick glucose 1 to 2 hours after eating. An alpha-glucosidase inhibitor such as acarbose or miglitol would be an appropriate choice in such patients because these agents work mainly by reducing the postprandial glucose value. If acarbose or miglitol is not tolerated, then a clinical trial of a thiazolidinedione, metformin, or low-dose glinides may be effective.

■ Nonobese Individuals With Diabetes

As mentioned earlier, thin patients may not respond as well to the oral agents as do obese patients. Lean patients with mild glucose intolerance can be given a trial with any of the four classes of oral agents, but sulfonylureas or glinides are likely to be a better initial choice for patients when blood glucose values are consistently in the 200 to 300 mg/dL range because these drugs can be titrated more rapidly to higher doses, which may be necessary in this patient group.

Late-onset type 1 diabetes should be considered in thin adults who do not respond well to oral agents. It is thought to occur in as many as 10% of "insulin-requiring type 2 diabetics," usually misdiagnosed as having type 2 diabetes because of their age. Because weeks to months can be wasted on unsuccessful trials of the various oral agents in this patient group, a blood test for glutamic acid decarboxylase (GAD) should be drawn and is indicative of type 1 diabetes. A fasting or meal-stimulated insulin or C-peptide level can also be obtained and is a simple method to assure the correct diagnosis and better direct treatment strategies (ie, insulin therapy) (see Chapter 8, *Insulin Therapy*).

■ Patients With Prolonged, Severe Hyperglycemia (Glucose Toxicity)

Ideally, a temporary trial of insulin therapy should be instituted for a few weeks before beginning an oral agent to reduce insulin resistance and improve endogenous insulin secretory capacity (see Chapter 8, *Insulin Therapy*). Improvement of metabolic control with insulin will increase the likelihood of a subsequent successful trial with an oral agent. Starting an oral agent when a patient has had prolonged and severe hyperglycemia is one of the most common causes of primary failure with an oral agent.

Another approach that has been used with some success is to start a sulfonylurea agent at the maximum dose and follow the patient carefully, usually with self monitoring of glucose. Once reasonable metabolic control is achieved with either insulin or maximum-dose sulfonylurea, the dosage requirements may fall as the glucose toxic state improves. At this point, switching to other oral agents with less hypoglycemic potential may be a reasonable alternative. Glinides may also be useful in this type of patient.

■ Patients With Severe Renal or Liver Dysfunction

Oral antidiabetic agents should be used with caution in patients with evidence of renal or liver disease (depending on the extent of organ dysfunction). In patients with renal impairment, alpha-glucosidase inhibitors are not absorbed systemically and may be used if mild-to-moderate glucose intolerance exists. Thiazolidinediones or glinides also represent excellent choices in this patient population since they are cleared almost entirely by the liver. These agents should not be initiated if evidence of active liver disease exists. In patients with significant or progressive liver disease, hyperglycemia is best treated with exogenous insulin alone.

Combination Therapy With Oral Antidiabetic Agents

The majority of patients with type 2 diabetes will not have adequate glycemic control with oral monotherapy. The reason a patient fails monotherapy is multifactorial, although the most common explanation is β-cell exhaustion, which reduces the response to oral agents. Combination therapy with two or more of the oral antidiabetic agents has been used extensively in many countries with excellent results and will

114

likely become the norm in the United States. This move to using more early combination therapy should enhance overall glycemic control and decrease diabetic complications. The different classes of oral antidiabetic agents are structurally and functionally unrelated (with the exception of sulfonylureas and glinides), and there are no known contraindications of using any of these agents in combination. Each of the different combinations has certain advantages and disadvantages for any given patient.

Taking Patients With Type 2 Diabetes Off Insulin

The availability of the new oral antidiabetic agents may enable some patients with type 2 diabetes to be taken off insulin. Clinical trials have demonstrated that when thiazolidinediones are added to insulin-requiring type 2 diabetics, there is improvement in glycemic control and a reduction in exogenous insulin requirements. Some patients may be able to come off insulin altogether. In general, if a patient is taking less than 40 to 50 units of insulin a day, then the success of achieving adequate control on oral agents alone is improved. Additional clinical characteristics that may indicate success in taking patients off insulin include:

- Duration of diabetes less than 10 years
- Overweight or obese individuals
- Absence of glucose toxicity, ie, fasting blood glucose values <200 mg/dL and/or postprandial blood glucose <250 mg/dL
- Diabetes diagnosed after age 35.

It is important to emphasize that these characteristics are only relative indications and should be used only as guidelines.

If a patient is on a combination of a daytime oral antidiabetic agent and bedtime insulin, then adding either a thiazolidinedione, metformin, or an alpha-glucosidase inhibitor during the day may prove effective in assisting the patient off insulin. When the new oral agent is started, the patient's insulin dose should be reduced by one third to one half, depending on the degree of glycemic control at the time of the attempted switchover. As the dose of the oral agent is increased, usually to the maximum dose, the insulin could be further reduced and eventually discontinued, depending on the home glucose readings.

In order to ensure safety, the patient should:
- Be reliable
- Be competent at home glucose monitoring
- Have ready telephone access to his/her caregiver.

Drugs Under Development

■ Amylin Analog

Amylin is a pancreatic β-cell hormone that is copackaged and cosecreted with insulin. Pramlintide is an analog of human amylin that has been shown to work by several different mechanisms including delaying the absorption of carbohydrates along the physiologic section of the GI tract and suppressing postprandial glucagon levels. Clinical trials in both type 1 and type 2 diabetes have demonstrated significant improvement in glycemic control while inducing weight loss which renders this injectable peptide potentially advantageous. Pramlintide is currently under development and will be marketed at Symlin.

■ Glucagon-like Peptide Analogs

Exendin-4 (Znalay) is a peptide first isolated from the oral secretions of the Gila monster which shares many properties of glucagon-like peptide (GLP)-1, especially in response to a meal. It has a much longer duration of action than GLP-1 and has many physiologic effects that improve the insulin resistant state. Synthetic exendin-4 has been studied in humans and has been shown to significantly lower postprandial glucose and triglyceride values, suppress glucagon, and slow gastric emptying. GLP-1 has also been shown to improve β-cell function in laboratory animals. It may also suppress appetite and lead to weight loss. GLP-1 analogs have the potential to make a major impact on the management of type 2 diabetes and the insulin-resistant syndrome.

SUGGESTED READING

American Diabetes Association. *Medical Management of Non–insulin-dependent (Type II) Diabetes*, 3rd ed. Alexandria, Va: American Diabetes Association; 1994:40-49.

Bakris GL, Dole JF, Porter LE, Huang C, Freed MI. Rosiglitazone improves blood pressure in patients with type 2 diabetes mellitus. *Diabetes*. 2000;49(suppl 1):A96. Abstract.

Buse J, Edelman SV, Neumann C. Precose resolution of optimal titration to enhance current therapies (P.R.O.T.E.C.T.) study: experience in patients with type II diabetes. *Diabetes*. 1997;46(suppl 1):A99. Abstract.

Chiasson JL, Josse RG, Hunt JA, et al. The efficacy of acarbose in the treatment of patients with non–insulin-dependent diabetes mellitus. *Ann Intern Med*. 1994;121: 928-935.

Cohen BR, Kreider M, Biswas N, Brunzell J, Ratner RE, Freed MI. Rosiglitazone in combination with an HMG CoA reductase inhibitor: safety and effects on lipid profile in patients with type 2 diabetes. *Diabetes*. 2001;50(suppl 2):A451. Abstract

Davidson J, Garber A, Mooradian A, Schneider S, Henry D. Metformin/glyburide tablets as first-line treatment in type 2 diabetes: distribution of HbA$_{1C}$ response. *Diabetes*. 2000;49(suppl 1):A356. Abstract.

DeFronzo RA, Goodman AM, The Multicenter Metformin Study Group. Efficacy of metformin in patients with non– insulin-dependent diabetes mellitus. *N Engl J Med*. 1995; 333:541-549.

7

Diabetes Control and Complications Trial Research Group. The effect of intensive treatment of diabetes on the development and progression of long-term complications in insulin-dependent diabetes mellitus. *N Engl J Med.* 1993;329: 977-986.

Edelman SV. Importance of glucose control. *Med Clin North Am.* 1998;82:665-687.

Egan JW, Lebrizzi R, Geerlof JS, et al. The long-term effect of pioglitazone as monotherapy or combination therapy on glucose control in patients with type 2 diabetes. *Diabetes.* 2000;49(suppl 1):A357. Abstract.

Egan JW, Mathisen AL, the Pioglitazone 012 Study Group. The effect of pioglitazone on glucose control and lipid profile in patients with type 2 diabetes. *Diabetes.* 2000;49(suppl 1):A105. Abstract.

Egan J, Rubin C, Mathisen A, the Pioglitazone 027 Study Group. Combination therapy with pioglitazone and metformin in patients with type 2 diabetes. *Diabetes.* 1999;48(suppl 1):A117. Abstract.

FDA Endocrinology and Metabolic Drug Advisory Committee; April 22th, 1999; on file with SmithKline Beecham Pharmaceuticals.

Fonseca V, Rosenstock J, Patwardhan R, Salzman A. Effect of metformin and rosiglitazone combination therapy in patients with type 2 diabetes mellitus: a randomized controlled trial. *JAMA.* 2000;283:1695-1702.

Freed M, Fuell D, Menci L, Heise M, Goldstein B. Effect of combination therapy with rosiglitazone and glibenclamide on PAI-1 antigen, PAI-1 activity, and tPA in patients with type 2 diabetes. *Diabetologia.* 2000;43(suppl 1):A267. Abstract.

Garber A. Davidson J, Mooradian A, Piper BA. Effect of metformin/glyburide tablets on HbA_{1C} in first-line treatment in type 2 diabetes. *Diabetes.* 2000;49(suppl 1):A364. Abstract.

Horton ES, Clinkingbeard C, Gatlin M, Foley J, Mallows S, Shen S. Nateglinide alone and in combination with metformin improves glycemic control by reducing mealtime glucose levels in type 2 diabetes. *Diabetes Care.* 2000;23:1660-1665.

Lebrizzi R, Egan JW, the Pioglitazone 010, 014, and 027 Study Groups. HbA$_{1C}$ and blood glucose response to pioglitazone in combination with another antidiabetic agent in patients with type 2 diabetes. *Diabetes*. 2000;49(suppl 1):A114. Abstract.

Mathisen A, Geerlof J, Houser V, the Pioglitazone 026 Study Group, Takeda America Research and Development Center, Inc. The effect of pioglitazone on glucose control and lipid profile in patients with type 2 diabetes. *Diabetes*. 1999;48(suppl 1):A102-A103. Abstract.

Mathisen A, Rubin C, et al. The long-term effect of pioglitazone on glucose control and lipid profile in patients with type 2 diabetes. *Diabetes*. 2000;49(suppl 1):A361-A362. Abstract.

Mohanty P, Aljada A, Ghanim H, et al. Rosiglitazone improves vascular reactivity, inhibits reactive oxygen species (ROS) generation, reduces p47phox subunit expression in mononuclear cells (MNC) and reduces C reactive protein (CRP) and monocyte chemotactic protein-1 (MCP-1): evidence of a potent anti-inflammatory effect. *Diabetes*. 2001;50(suppl 2):A68. Abstract.

Patel JAI, Miller E, Patwardham R, the Rosiglitazone Study Group. Rosiglitazone (BRL49653) monotherapy has significant glucose lowering effect in type 2 diabetic patients. *Diabetes*. 1998;47(suppl 1):A17. Abstract.

Porter LE, Freed MI, Jones NP, Biswas N. Rosiglitazone improves β-cell function as measured by proinsulin/insulin ratio in patients with type 2 diabetes. *Diabetes*. 2000;49(suppl 1):A122. Abstract.

Reichard P, Nilsson BY, Rosenqvist U. The effect of long-term intensified insulin treatment on the development of microvascular complications of diabetes mellitus. *N Engl J Med*. 1993;329:304-309.

Rosenstock J, Donavan D, Piper BA. Effect of metformin/glyburide tablets on postprandial insulin as first-line in type 2 diabetes. *Diabetes*. 2000;49(suppl 1):A364. Abstract.

Rubin C, Egan JW, the Pioglitazone 010, 014, and 027 Study Groups. HbA$_{1C}$ and blood glucose response to pioglitazone in combination with another antidiabetic agent in patients with type 2 diabetes. *Diabetes*. 2000;49(suppl 1):A114. Abstract.

7

Schneider R, Egan J, Schjneider R, the Pioglitazone 010 Study Group. Combination therapy with sulfonylurea in patients with type 2 diabetes. *Diabetes*. 1999;48(suppl 1):A106. Abstract.

Shaffer S, Rubin C, Zhu E. The effect of pioglitazone lipid profile in patients with type 2 diabetes. *Diabetes*. 2000; 49(suppl 1):A125. Abstract.

Sutton MSJ, Dole JF, Rappaport EB. Rosiglitazone does not adversely affect cardiac structure or function in patients with type 2 diabetes. *Diabetes*. 1999;48(suppl 1);A102. Abstract 0438.

United Kingdom Prospective Diabetes Study (UKPDS) Group. Intensive blood-glucose control with sulphonylureas or insulin compared with conventional treatment and risk complications in patients with type 2 diabetes (UKPDS 33). *Lancet*. 1998;352:837-853.

Wolffenbuttel BH, Gomis R, Squatrito S, Jones NP, Patwardhan RN. Addition of low-dose rosiglitazone to sulphonylurea therapy improves glycaemic control in type 2 diabetic patients. *Diabetic Med*. 2000;17:40-47.

8   Insulin Therapy

Insulin therapy most commonly is reserved for patients who have failed an adequate trial of diet, exercise, and oral antidiabetic agents. However, institution of insulin therapy is commonly delayed inappropriately for months to years in patients failing oral antidiabetic agents. Both physicians and patients are hesitant to start "the needle" because of fear, ignorance, and time constraints. There is no question that the benefits of improved glycemic control outweigh the hassles and risks of insulin therapy. We encourage early use of insulin soon after it is evident that oral antidiabetic agents are failing.

Many insulin regimens are recommended, although it is not clear from the literature which regimen is best. This chapter will focus on the different insulin regimens commonly used to normalize glucose levels and glycosylated hemoglobin (HbA_{1C}) in patients with type 2 diabetes mellitus.

Based on the natural history of type 2 diabetes, many patients will eventually require therapy with insulin. The period of time before insulin is required tends to be highly variable and is based on numerous factors. The most important explanation is the extent of β-cell exhaustion resulting in relative endogenous insulinopenia. This leads to progressive loss of compensatory hyperinsulinemia, which is required to achieve and maintain a sufficient degree of glycemic control, especially in patients taking oral hypoglycemic agents. In other cases, obesity, pregnancy, or any number of medications, as well as a variety of medical illnesses, may exacerbate the insulin-resistant state and convert a patient previously well controlled on oral agents to one requiring insulin.

In addition to the natural history of type 2 diabetes, there is heterogeneity in its pathophysiology, which may influence when patients require insulin. Some patients diagnosed with type 2 diabetes may actually be closer to insulin-dependent or type 1 diabetes with severe insulinopenia. Many of these patients have been shown to have islet cell antibody (ICA) positivity or antibodies to glutamic acid decarboxylase (GAD), with a decreased C-peptide response to glucagon stimulation and a propensity for primary oral medication failure. There are also wide geographic and racial differences that may influence the need for insulin therapy. For example, Asian patients with type 2 diabetes tend to be thinner, to be diagnosed with diabetes at an earlier age, to fail oral hypoglycemic agents much sooner, and to be more sensitive to insulin therapy than the classic centrally obese Caucasian patient.

Insulin therapy can improve or correct many of the metabolic abnormalities present in patients with type 2 diabetes mellitus. Exogenous insulin administration significantly reduces glucose levels by suppressing hepatic glucose production, increasing postprandial glucose utilization, and improving the abnormal lipoprotein levels commonly seen in patients with insulin resistance. Insulin therapy may also decrease or eliminate the effects of glucose toxicity by reducing hyperglycemia to improve insulin sensitivity and beta cell secretory function.

Selecting an Insulin Preparation

The three types of insulin are animal, human, and insulin analogs. Purified insulins are available, including beef and pork, although human insulin is the predominant form used. In addition, insulin lispro (Humalog) and aspart (Novolog) are fast-acting insulin analogs available for clinical use (Figure 8.1). In-

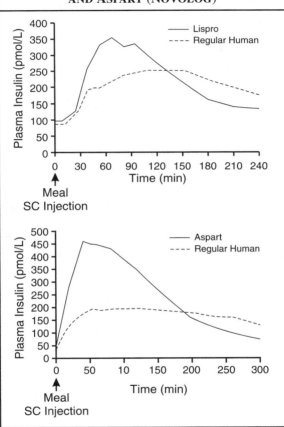

FIGURE 8.1 — FAST-ACTING INSULIN ANALOGS: LISPRO (HUMALOG) AND ASPART (NOVOLOG)

Abbreviation: SC, subcutaneous.

Heinemann, et al. *Diabet Med*. 1996;13:625-629; Mudaliar, et al. *Diabetes Care*. 1999;22:1501-1506.

sulin preparations available to control blood glucose in patients with type 2 diabetes mellitus include:

- Fast-acting insulin (lispro, aspart)
- Short-acting preparations (regular insulin),
- Intermediate-acting insulins (NPH, lente insulins)
- Ultra long-acting insulins (ultralente, glargine insulins).

The fast-acting insulin analogs are preferential to regular insulin due to their favorable clinical features. Administration is convenient as they can be given immediately prior to or with meals. Their faster onset of action limits postprandial hyperglycemic peaks by matching serum insulin availability to appearance of meal-derived glucose into the circulation. Their shorter duration of action also reduces development of late postprandial hypoglycemia. The analogs are used to control postprandial glucose and need to be given in concert with basal insulin replacement regimens.

Short/fast-acting insulins, as well as long-acting insulin preparations, are needed to mimic the pattern of insulin delivery that normally controls blood glucose in nondiabetic individuals. Basal insulin therapy with long-acting insulin is required to suppress hepatic glucose production overnight and between meals, while short/rapid insulin preparations are needed as bolus insulin to prevent hyperglycemia after meals.

Human insulin is particularly useful for patients with:

- Insulin allergy
- Severe insulin resistance caused by insulin antibodies
- Lipoatrophy
- A requirement for intermittent insulin therapy (ie, during pregnancy and acute problems such

as infection, myocardial infarction, and emergency surgery).

Many of the complications of insulin therapy are now uncommon because of the advent of more purified human preparations.

Selecting an appropriate insulin preparation also depends on the desired time course of action or pharmacokinetics. The values shown in Table 8.1 are general guidelines that can vary considerably among individuals, especially those with type 2 diabetes. Other factors that influence the action of insulin within an individual include:

- Site and depth of injection
- Local tissue blood blow
- Skin temperature
- Exercise.

The time courses of action of the various insulins are shown graphically in Figure 8.2. The recommended interval between an injection of regular or fast-acting insulins and mealtime is 30 to 45 and 5 minutes, respectively, when the preprandial blood glucose is adequate (less than 140 mg/dL). The patient should wait longer if the blood glucose is higher. Proper timing of the premeal injection can markedly improve the postprandial blood glucose level and possibly reduce the incidence of delayed hypoglycemia (Figure 10.3). Eating within a few minutes of the injection, or before the injection of regular insulin, markedly reduces the ability of the insulin to prevent a rapid rise in blood glucose and may increase the risk of delayed hypoglycemia. Humalog and Novolog have alleviated much of this problem because of their rapid onset and short duration of activity. Common insulin regimens used in adult diabetes are listed in Table 8.2.

8

TABLE 8.1 — TIME COURSE OF ACTION OF INSULIN PREPARATIONS

Insulin Preparation	Onset of Action	Peak Action	Duration of Action
Mealtime Insulins			
Short-acting (regular)	30 min	2-5 h	5-8 h
Fast-acting (Lispro–Humalog or Aspart–Novolog)*	Minutes	<1 hour	3-5 h
Basal Insulins			
Intermediate-acting (NPH or Lente)	1-3 h	6-8 h	16-24 h
Long-acting (Ultralente)	Gradual	8-20 h	24-28 h
Glargine (Lantus)*	Gradual	Peakless	24 hr
Fixed Mixtures			
Humalog Mix75/25*	Minutes	7-12 h	16-24 h
Human (70/30, 50/50)	30 min	7-12 h	16-24 h
Abbreviation: NPH, neutral protamine Hagedorn.			

This table summarizes the typical time course of action of various insulin preparations. Values are highly variable among individuals; in a given patient, these values vary depending on the site and depth of injection, local tissue blood flow, skin temperature, and exercise.

* Reproducibility of time course of action and efficacy may be improved with insulin analogs.

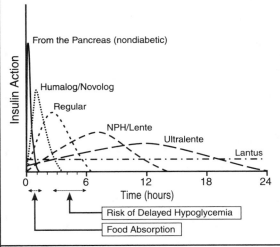

FIGURE 8.2 — PEAK ACTION OF INSULIN COMPARED WITH PEAK RISE IN GLUCOSE AFTER EATING

The time course of action (pharmacokinetics) for the fast-acting insulin analogs *(dotted line)* is not as fast as insulin from the pancreas of a nondiabetic individual *(solid line),* but it is much more physiologic than the older Regular insulin preparations *(short-dashed line).* Also shown is the time course of action of the intermediate- and long-acting insulins, including the new long-acting insulin analog glargine.

Application of Intensive Insulin Therapy

The goals of therapy should be individually tailored. Candidates for intensive management should be:
- Motivated
- Compliant
- Educable

TABLE 8.2 — COMMON INSULIN REGIMENS USED IN ADULT DIABETES

Regimen	Administration	Comment
Single-injection insulin	NPH or Lente alone or with Humalog/Novolog or regular insulin at breakfast, supper, or bedtime, depending on HGM results	Glucose control usually inadequate with single-injection therapy
Insulin and oral agents	Glargine, NPH, or Lente at bedtime or premixed 70/30 or Humalog Mix75/25 before supper added to oral antidiabetic agents	Total oral dose of the antidiabetic agents can be given before breakfast if predinner blood glucose values remain elevated
Multiple-injection insulin	Glargine, NPH, Lente, or Ultralente with regular insulin prebreakfast and supper; regular or Humalog/Novolog insulin before meals; and NPH, Lente or Ultralente at bedtime or late afternoon	Premixed Human 70/30 or Humalog Mix75/25 prebreakfast and predinner is useful, especially in obese patients with high insulin requirements
Pump therapy insulin	Novolog or Humalog insulin given as bolus and basal rates	Effective strategy for patients with inflexible work hours and/or who are not doing well on a conventional insulin regimen

Abbreviations: NPH, neutral protamine Hagedorn; HGM, home glucose monitoring.

- Without other medical conditions and physical limitations that preclude accurate and reliable self-monitoring of blood glucose (SMBG) and insulin administration.

In addition, caution is advised in patients who are elderly or who are unaware of the signs of hypoglycemia. Other limitations to achieving normoglycemia may include high titers of insulin antibodies, especially in those patients with a prior history of intermittent insulin use of animal origin. The site of insulin injection may also change the pharmacokinetics, and absorption can be highly variable, especially if lipohypertrophy is present. The periumbilical area has been shown to be one of the most desirable areas to inject insulin because of the rapid and consistent absorption kinetics observed at this location.

Prior to initiating insulin therapy, the patient should be well educated in the:

- Techniques of SMBG
- Proper techniques of mixing insulins and administration
- Self adjustment of insulin dose if appropriate
- Dietary and exercise strategies.

The patient and family members also need to be informed about hypoglycemia prevention, recognition, and treatment. Initial and ongoing education by a diabetes management team is crucial for long-term success and safety.

Combination Therapy

Combination therapy usually refers to the use of oral antidiabetic agents (daytime) together with a single injection of intermediate-acting or long-acting insulin at bedtime. The rationale for using an evening insulin strategy is based on the pathophysiology of fasting hyperglycemia in type 2 diabetes. The underlying tenet for combination therapy assumes that if evening insulin lowers the fasting glucose level to normal levels, then the daytime oral agent will be more effective at controlling postprandial hyperglycemia and maintaining euglycemia throughout the day. Metabolic profiles in type 2 diabetes have clearly demonstrated that the fasting blood glucose is a major determinant or predictor of glycemic control throughout the day. The fasting blood glucose level is highly correlated with the degree of hepatic glucose production during the early morning hours, which is suppressed by bedtime insulin. In addition, bedtime intermediate-acting insulin's peak action coincides with the onset of the dawn phenomenon (early morning resistance to insulin caused by diurnal variations in growth hormone and possibly norepinephrine levels), which usually occurs between 3:00 and 7:00 AM.

Patient selection is very important when considering combination therapy. The question of whether a patient is still responding in a satisfactory manner to oral antidiabetic agent(s), such as sulfonylureas, is of primary importance. Patients also have a higher likelihood of success using daytime oral agents and bedtime insulin if they:

- Are obese
- Have had overt diabetes for less than 10 to 15 years
- Are diagnosed with type 2 diabetes after the age of 35
- Do not have fasting blood glucose values consistently over 250 to 300 mg/dL
- Have evidence of endogenous insulin secretory ability.

Although standard measurement conditions and levels for C-peptide have not been established for this clinical situation, a fasting (0.2 nmol/L or 0.6 ng/mL) or glucagon-stimulated (>0.40 nmol/L or 1.2 ng/mL) C-peptide value indicates some degree of endogenous insulin secretory ability. Patients with type 2 diabetes diagnosed under the age of 35 more often have atypical forms of diabetes. Subjects with diabetes longer than 10 to 15 years in duration tend to have a greater chance of β-cell exhaustion and thus be less responsive to the oral antidiabetic agents.

Thin patients are more likely to be hypoinsulinemic and often respond inadequately to oral sulfonylureas, which leads to combination-therapy failure. In addition, when the fasting glucose level becomes markedly elevated, this is often associated with a concomitant decrease in endogenous insulin secretory ability, which renders oral agents less effective. The actual number of patients who might fit into this category and possibly respond to combination therapy is unknown but is estimated to be between 20% and 30% of all patients "failing" maximum doses of oral agent therapy.

There are also a number of practical reasons why combination therapy may be beneficial (Table 8.2):

- The patient does not need to learn how to mix different types of insulin
- Hospitalization is not required
- Patient compliance and acceptance are better with single rather than multiple injections of insulin
- The patient does not need to take injections during the day while at work or other activities
- Enables the patient to be initiated on insulin in a simple straightforward manner.

Combination therapy also requires a lower total dose of exogenous insulin than a full two- or three-injection-a-day regimen. This usually contributes to less weight gain and peripheral hyperinsulinemia.

Calculation of the initial bedtime intermediate-acting insulin dose can be based on clinical judgment or on various formulas using fasting blood glucose level or body weight. For example, one can divide the average fasting blood glucose (mg/dL) by 18 or divide the body weight in kilograms by 10 to calculate the initial dose of NPH, Lente, or glargine to be started at bedtime. One can also safely start 5 to 10 units of intermediate-acting or long-acting insulin (NPH, Lente, or glargine) for thin patients and 10 to 15 units for obese patients at bedtime as an initial estimated dose. In either case, the dose is increased in 2 to 5 unit increments every 3 to 4 days until the morning fasting blood glucose level is consistently in the range of 80 to 140 mg/dL (Table 8.3).

TABLE 8.3 — GUIDELINES FOR DOSING INSULIN IN COMBINATION THERAPY

1. To calculate insulin dose (NPH, Lente, or glargine): divide average fasting blood glucose (mg/dL) by 18 or divide body weight (kg) by 10 to calculate initial dose of NPH or Lente insulin for bedtime (10:00 PM to midnight).

2. Initial bedtime dose for lean patients: 5-10 U intermediate-acting insulin.

3. Initial bedtime dose for obese patients: 10-15 U intermediate-acting insulin.

4. Increase dose of insulin in increments of 2-5 U every 3-4 days until the AM fasting blood glucose level is consistently 70-140 mg/dL (reliable patients can make their own adjustments using results from home glucose monitoring).

5. Patients continue taking the maximum dose of their oral agents; if daytime glucose levels become too low (<100 mg/dL), the dose of the oral agent must be decreased.

6. If the oral agent cannot maintain daytime euglycemia, other oral agents can be used or conventional insulin therapy started.

Abbreviation: NPH, neutral protamine Hagedorn.

The most ideal time to give the evening injection of intermediate-acting or long-acting insulin is between 10 PM and midnight. Many reliable patients can make their own adjustments using SMBG. Table 8.4 demonstrates a patient self-instruction sheet for bedtime insulin adjustments. Once the fasting blood glucose levels are consistently in a desirable range, the prelunch, predinner, and bedtime blood glucose must be monitored to determine if the oral hypoglycemic agents are maintaining daytime euglycemia.

TABLE 8.4 — PATIENT SELF ADJUSTMENT OF EVENING INSULIN

1. Begin with a dose of _____ units of _____ insulin administered just before bedtime (NPH, Lente, Glargine).

2. If the prebreakfast blood sugar is >140 mg/dL for 3 days in a row, then increase the evening _____ insulin dose by _____ units.

3. If the prebreakfast blood sugar is <80 mg/dL for 2 days in a row, then decrease the evening insulin by _____ units.

4. Remember not to increase the insulin dose more frequently than every 3 days.

5. If you have any questions, please call me at _____.

6. Provider's name:_____.

_____
Physician/Nurse Practitioner

Based on the results of SMBG, combination therapy can be altered to reduce hyperglycemia at identified times during the day. For example, a common situation seen with daytime sulfonylureas and bedtime intermediate-acting or long-acting insulin is an improvement in the fasting, prelunch, and predinner blood glucose, although the postdinner blood glucose level remains excessively high (>200 mg/dL). In this clinical situation, an injection of premixed regular and intermediate-acting insulin (ie, Humalog Mix75/25 insulin) predinner instead of the bedtime dose of intermediate-acting insulin may be more efficacious. This regimen will often improve the postdinner blood glucose values, because the premixed insulin contains rapidly acting regular insulin yet will still allow overnight glucose control secondary to the intermediate-acting component. With this regimen, however, one must be more cautious of early morning hypoglycemia because the intermediate insulin given before dinner will exert its peak effect earlier. This latter concern has not been a major clinical problem in patients with type 2 diabetes compared with those with type 1 diabetes mellitus.

It is recommended that after addition of evening insulin, patients remain on their maximal dose of oral antidiabetic agent. If the daytime blood glucose levels start to become excessively low, the dose of oral medication must be adjusted downward. This is not an uncommon scenario because glucose toxicity may be reduced as a result of improved glucose control, leading to enhanced sensitivity to both oral agents and insulin. If the prelunch and predinner blood glucose levels remain excessively high on combination therapy, the oral antidiabetic agent is likely not contributing significantly to glycemic control throughout the day. In this situation, use of other oral antidiabetic can be utilized or a more conventional two-injection-a-day regimen can be employed while discontinuing the oral antidiabetic agents.

In summary, combination therapy can be a simple and effective tool to normalize glycemia and HbA_{1C} levels in selected patients with type 2 diabetes mellitus failing oral antidiabetic agents. The most common clinical situation where combination therapy can be successful is in the patient failing oral antidiabetic therapy but with some evidence of responsiveness to the oral agents. Bedtime intermediate-acting or long-acting insulin is given and progressively increased so as to normalize the fasting blood glucose level. When the fasting blood glucose level is brought under control, the success of combination therapy is dependent on the ability of the daytime oral antidiabetic agents to maintain euglycemia. If this cannot be achieved, then other oral antidiabetic agents can be used or conventional insulin regimens employed.

Multiple Injection Regimens

One of the most common insulin regimens utilized in type 2 diabetes mellitus is a split-mixed regimen consisting of a prebreakfast and predinner dose of an intermediate- and fast-acting insulin. This split-mixed two-injection-a-day regimen is often inadequate for patients with type 1 diabetes mellitus and results in persistent early morning hypoglycemia and fasting hyperglycemia. Such problems do not appear to occur as frequently in type 2 diabetes. This is likely because of pathophysiologic differences between type 1 and type 2 diabetes, particularly in:
- Endogenous insulin secretory ability
- Insulin resistance
- Counterregulatory mechanisms.

There are a number of important aspects about intensive glucose control with insulin in obese patients with type 2 diabetes:
- First, the average daily dose of insulin needed to aggressively control such patients may approximate one unit per kilogram of body weight.
- Second, the total daily insulin requirement can successfully be split equally between the prebreakfast and predinner injections.

- Third, obese patients will require approximately 70% of their total insulin requirement as NPH or Lente with the remainder as a mealtime insulin, such as Humalog, Novolog, or regular insulin.
- Fourth, the split-mixed regimen in obese patients with type 2 diabetes is usually devoid of the common problems seen with this regimen in type 1 diabetes, particularly early morning hypoglycemia and fasting (preprandial) hyperglycemia.
- Fifth, mild and severe hypoglycemic events are much less frequent in patients with type 2 diabetes mellitus compared with patients with type 1 diabetes undergoing intensive insulin therapy.
- Sixth, the use of fast-acting insulin analogs such as Humalog and Novolog instead of the older regular insulins may be helpful in terms of reducing prolonged postprandial hyperglycemia, glycosylated hemoglobin, and the incidence of delayed hypoglycemia.
- Finally, weight gain with peripheral hyperinsulinemia frequently occurs in type 2 diabetes when glucose control is intensified with insulin therapy.

In most cases, single-injection therapy with an intermediate- or long-acting insulin has been shown to be inadequate to normalize glycosylated hemoglobin and maintain 24-hour euglycemia in type 2 diabetes.

There are several acceptable methods to initiate insulin therapy in type 2 diabetes. A conservative yet effective strategy utilizing a step-wise approach to instituting a split-mixed regimen is given in Table 8.5. A simple alternative method to initiating a split-mixed regimen in obese patients uses 70/30 or 75/25 premixed insulin with an initial total daily insulin dose

TABLE 8.5 — STEPWISE APPROACH FOR INITIATING A SPLIT-MIXED INSULIN REGIMEN IN PATIENTS WITH TYPE 2 DIABETES

1. **First Goal**: **fasting BG 80 mg/dL to 120 mg/dL**
   Initial dose of NPH or Lente insulin: 0.2 U/kg before dinner.
   Change dose of evening NPH insulin based on subsequent fasting BG as follows:
   - If BG >180 mg/dL, increase by 0.5 U/kg
   - If BG 120 mg/dL to 180 md/dL, increase by 0.05 U/kg
   - If BG 80 mg/dL to 120 mg/dL, no change in dose
   - If BG <80 mg/dL, decrease by 0.1 U/kg.

2. **Second Goal**: **predinner BG 80 mg/dL to 120 mg/dL**
   Initial dose of NPH or Lente insulin before breakfast and criteria for adjustment same as for first goal, except based on subsequent predinner BG.
   Proceed to third goal only after first and second goals are achieved.

3. **Third Goal**: **postprandial (1-2 h) BG <180 md/dL (after breakfast and dinner)**
   Change each dose of Humalog or Novolog insulin based on subsequent postprandial (1-2 h) BG as follows:
   - If BG >180 mg/dL, increase by 0.025 U/kg
   - If BG 120 mg/dL to 180 mg/dL, no change in dose
   - If BG 80 mg/dL to 120 mg/dL, decrease by 0.025 U/kg
   - If BG <80 mg/dL increase dose by 0.05 U/kg

   All injections should be given subcutaneously in the periumbilical region 5 to 15 minutes before breakfast and dinner.

Abbreviations: BG, blood glucose; U, units.

Source: Adapted from Henry RR, Edelman SV. Metabolic disorders. Diabetes mellitus in adults. In: Rakel RE, ed. *Conn's Current Therapy*. Philadelphia, Pa: WB Saunders Co; 1996:526.

8

(0.4 to 0.8 units/kg) equally split between the prebreakfast and predinner injections. Adjustments are made based on SMBG results, which may dictate the need to change the ratio of intermediate- to regular-acting insulin either upward or downward. For morbidly obese patients, the insulin requirements rise dramatically as ideal body weight increases above 150%. In contrast, caution should be used when starting thin patients with type 2 diabetes on insulin, especially premixed insulins with fixed doses of regular insulin (total daily dose 0.2 to 0.5 units/kg). This group tends to be more sensitive to the glucose-lowering effects and thus more prone to severe hypoglycemia. If a multiple injection regimen or insulin pump is to be initiated, then the basal insulin requirements (ie, Ultralente or Glargine for the multiple injection regimens) should be 50% to 60% of the total daily insulin requirements. The remainder of the total dose should be in boluses premeals in the form of a fast-acting insulin analog (Humalog or Novalog). Premeal boluses of regular or lispro insulin are also given with adjustment based on the 1- to 2-hour postprandial blood glucose measurements.

In summary, there is no one perfect insulin regimen that can be used in type 2 diabetes. In a subgroup of patients failing maximum doses of sulfonylureas or other oral agents, combination therapy can be beneficial, easy to administer, and reduce the need for large doses of exogenous insulin.

Insulin Pump Therapy

Insulin pump therapy has been traditionally used for people with type 1 diabetes. People with type 1 diabetes usually do not have insulin resistance, therefore, they require low basal rates and small insulin boluses. Because type 2 diabetics have the underlying defect of insulin resistance in addition to β-cell failure, they have increased insulin requirements. Insulin pump therapy is extremely valuable in patients with insulin-requiring type 2 diabetes who have not achieved glycemic control with subcutaneous injections, who are experiencing wide fluctuations in blood glucose levels complicated by hypoglycemia, or who are seeking a more flexible lifestyle. All of the benefits that are enjoyed by patients with type 1 diabetes discussed previously also apply to people with type 2 diabetes. There are other potential advantages to pump therapy. A patient with type 2 diabetes should be treated with the minimal amount of insulin possible to improve glucose control because excess insulin administration could cause further weight gain. When the pump is used, the number of hypoglycemic events decreases. Therefore, there is less overeating to compensate for hypoglycemia and weight gain may be less of an issue.

Many older patients with the diagnosis of insulin requiring type 2 diabetes have true late onset type 1 diabetes. It has been documented in the literature that when large groups of patients with insulin-requiring type 2 diabetes mellitus were tested for anti-gluamic acid decarboxylase (GAD) antibodies, approximately 5% to 8% are positive. These individuals are thinner at the time of diagnosis, generally do not respond well to oral agents, and require insulin, although they do not present in severe diabetic ketoacidosis. This is another group that could potentially benefit from insulin pump therapy. In general, if a patient with insulin-requiring type 2 diabetes cannot achieve glycemic control with an intensive insulin injection regimen, then insulin pump therapy should be considered.

New Types of Insulin Preparations

■ Insulin Lispro

Lispro (Humalog) is a relatively new type of regular (or fast-acting) insulin. Patients with insulin-requiring diabetes in the general population have now used it safely and effectively for the past several years. It is an effective agent for improving glycemic control while minimizing delayed hypoglycemia. The rapid onset of action appears to be mainly due to its faster absorption (peaking at approximately 30 to 60 minutes as compared with 60 to 120 minutes for regular insulin) when injected subcutaneously. Its unique absorption and action properties are the result of a reversal in the two adjacent amino acids: lysine at position 28 and proline at position 29 on the β-chain.

Some of the drawbacks of the older regular insulin preparations have been their slow onset of action as well as delayed clearance resulting in inefficient control of postprandial excursions in blood glucose levels. With the faster rise and fall of serum insulin level following a lispro injection, it is easier to coordinate the timing of insulin injections with the subsequent meal. Another advantage to this fact-acting insulin is that it does not have as prolonged an action as the currently available regular insulin, thereby reducing the incidence of delayed hypoglycemic reactions.

Insulin lispro has also been made available recently in a premixed formulation called Humalog Mix75/25. This form of insulin contains 75% of an intermediate-acting insulin called neutral protamine lispro, or the NPL component, and 25% of insulin lispro. Because of the rapid onset of activity of this new mixture, it can be given anytime within 15 minutes before a meal, yet it has a duration of activity similar to 70/30. This new mixture is available at this time only in a prefilled syringe.

140

The benefits of using a mixture of insulin lispro and NPL include:

- Use of lispro which is effective in reducing postprandial hyperglycemia
- No need to mix insulin lispro and NPH in separate syringes
- No need to wait 30 to 45 minutes between an injection and mealtime
- Dosing accuracy is improved in a pen compared with a syringe
- A lowered incidence of delayed hypoglycemia with the shorter-acting lispro in the mixture.

Patients with type 2 diabetes new to insulin might be considered good candidates for this new mixture. In addition, patients already on 70/30, NPH insulin alone, or oral agents but who remain out of control or who have delayed hypoglycemia may benefit from this mixture.

■ Insulin Aspart

Insulin aspart (Novolog) is another fast-acting insulin analog recently developed by substituting proline with aspartate on the beta chain of the insulin molecule. This insulin will be much more quickly absorbed than regular insulin with similar benefits as lispro. It has recently completed final stages of clinical trials and has been approved for therapeutic use in insulin-requiring diabetics.

■ Insulin Glargine

Insulin glargine (Lantus) is the first true peakless long-acting basal insulin analog. Produced by recombinant DNA technology, it differs from human insulin through a change in one amino acid on the insulin A chain and two amino acids on the B chain. It exists in an acidic form and cannot be mixed in the same syringe with other insulins. After subcutaneous injection, insulin glargine forms microcrystalline precipitates that gradually release insulin. Glargine has its onset of action at 4 to 6 hours and a duration of action of more than 24 hours without a peak. The rate of absorption does not differ for different injection sites and the pharmacokinetics within subjects are fairly consistent.

Initial studies in patients with both type 1 and type 2 diabetes mellitus have shown that the drug is effective when either regular insulin or insulin lispro is used as adjunctive mealtime insulin. Glargine is also being studied as an additive agent to patients with type 2 diabetes taking oral agents. The Treat to Target study is comparing the effects of NPH or glargine at bedtime in patients failing oral agents. Although the study is still in progress and the two groups are not yet unblinded, the combined data demonstrate an impressive reduction in glycosylated HbA_{1C} from 8.5% to 6.9% in just 15 weeks. To date, the average insulin dose is approximately 45 units and the subjects have only gained 3.3 lbs. Listed below are several clinical suggestions for glargine usage.

Switching a Patient From the Traditional Split-Mixed Regimen to Glargine

The recommended change over suggests that the total NPH or Lente dose be reduced by 20% to determine the nighttime dose of glargine. It is important, however, to remember that a fast-acting insulin should be used before each meal, including lunch, with this new regimen. The total amount of insulin on the new glargine/fast-acting insulin regimen should approximate the total split-mixed regimen dose. An example would be a 29-year-old white male who is taking 15 units of NPH and 5 to 10 units of Humalog or Novolog before breakfast and 10 units of NPH and 5 to 10 units of Humalog or Novolog before dinner. We recommend starting with an initial glargine dose of approximately 20 units at bedtime but also add in a prelunch injection of Humalog or Novolog of 5 to 10 units. Further adjustments should be based on the results of premeal and postmeal home glucose monitoring.

Switching a Patient From an Ultralente Twice a Day Plus Fast-Acting Insulin Regimen (Multiple Daily Injections) to Glargine

In this scenario, the conversion is slightly easier. Take the total ultralente dose and subtract either 0% to 5% to get the initial glargine dose. If the HbA_{1C} value is fairly good on the Ultralente regimen, then subtract 5% and if the degree of control is not adequate, then use the total Ultralente dose to calculate the glargine dose. The premeal doses of Humalog or Novolog that are being used would be the same.

When Converting a Patient From an Insulin Pump (Patients With Type 2 Diabetes are Candidates for an Insulin Pump) to a Glargine Regimen or Vice Versa

We would take the amount of insulin used for the basal rate of the pump and use that for the initial glargine dose and vice versa when initiating pump therapy from a glargine/fast-acting insulin regimen. In our experience, we have achieved fairly good success with using similar total doses without any reductions. Obviously, the premeal dose of Humalog or Novolog does not change when converting to this regimen. On the first night of the glargine injection when initiating pump therapy, we ask the patient to take the dose of glargine earlier in the evening, ie, 5 or 6 PM, and continued the basal rate of the pump until bedtime in order to avoid hyperglycemia the next morning.

Other Issues Regarding the Use of Glargine

It is recommended that glargine be taken at bedtime although it can be taken at any time that it is convenient for the patient. A patient who goes from an insulin pump to a glargine regimen may forget to take the injection of glargine at night during the first few weeks after initiating therapy leading to morning hyperglycemia. Methods to avoid forgetting should be implemented such as leaving a note or some type or reminder near the bedside clock or nightstand.

Glargine can cause burning when injected although we have not found this to be a problem.

Occasionally, a patient may state that he or she feels that glargine has a peak and is causing hypoglycemia to develop approximately 12 hours after injecting. If this is true, the time of injection can be changed and the home glucose monitoring data should be reviewed after several days.

In patients using large doses of glargine (ie, >30 to 50 units/day), it may be beneficial to split the dose of glargine in the morning and in the evening although this has not been documented in clinical trials.

Alternative Insulin Delivery Systems

A recent publication indicates that the inhaled form of insulin in type 2 diabetes mellitus is quickly absorbed, very similar to the pharmacokinetics of the rapid-acting analogs. Inhaled insulin have also demonstrated reproducible pharmacologic effects on blood glucose, similar to those of subcutaneously (SC) injected rapid-acting insulin, and is generally well tolerated. Pulmonary safety surveillance studies are ongoing in healthy individuals with diabetes mellitus as well as asthmatics and smokers. Safety data including pulmonary function testing for up to 36 months have been analyzed without findings of major adverse events.

Nasal and aerosolized oral insulins, which may also have better pharmacokinetic properties than SC insulin, are currently being tested in phase 2 and 3 trials.

Complications of Insulin Therapy

Weight gain and hypoglycemia are the most frequently reported complications of insulin therapy. Both can be minimized with appropriate preventive measures and dosage adjustments. It is important to emphasize that the benefits of improved glycemic control far outweigh any adverse effects of weight gain in a patient with poorly controlled diabetes.

■ Weight Gain

Hyperinsulinemia caused by large amounts of exogenous insulin can lead to marked increases in weight, which is a real concern in type 2 diabetes. Obesity itself is an insulin-resistant state that contributes to a cycle of worsening insulin resistance, increasing insulin requirements, and further weight gain. Some patients, particularly the obese, may require large doses of insulin to normalize glycemia in order to overcome the insulin resistance that is typical of type 2 diabetes. The additional exogenous insulin can result in hyperinsulinemia and an average increase in body weight of 3% to 9%. Excessive weight gain can be minimized by using the lowest possible dose of insulin to achieve target glycemic goals and encouraging the patient to decrease caloric intake and increase exercise.

■ Hypoglycemia

The incidence of hypoglycemic reaction increases with insulin therapy, particularly intensive regimens, and the thin and the elderly are most affected by such episodes. Obese patients with type 2 diabetes tend to have much less hypoglycemia than those with type 1 diabetes. Severe hypoglycemia is rare in obese patients with type 2 diabetes and is usually related to causal factors such as:

- Overinsulinization
- Underfeeding
- Unplanned strenuous physical activity
- Excessive alcohol
- Incorrect dose of insulin or oral agents taken by patient.

Frequent SMBG by the patient with adjustment in the dose or type of insulin can significantly reduce the likelihood of hypoglycemia.

Islet Cell Transplantation

Islet cell transplantation is an exciting area of investigation that may some day become the forefront of diabetes treatment. Most of the research has been performed in laboratory animals; human trials have been limited to people with type 1 diabetes with end-stage renal disease (status-post or in need of renal transplant) who require immunosuppressive therapy. Currently, islet cell transplantation is indicated for patients who have had a total pancreatectomy for chronic pancreatitis (islet autograft transplantation) or in patients with type 1 diabetes (islet allograft). Some of the major problems have been in harvesting and preserving sufficient numbers of islet cells while avoiding the damaging effects of the surrounding enzyme-producing digestive cells of the exocrine pancreas. Techniques such as islet encapsulation, cryopreservation, and xenographs from foreign species are currently being developed to prevent immune rejection of transplanted islet cells and enhance long-term therapeutic effectiveness. Islet cell transplantation is associated with a 2-year pancreatic function survival rate of about 80%. Islet allograft transplantation, however, has had very limited success. Newer and more effective anti-rejection drugs with lower side effects such as FK 506 have also helped improve graft survival rates.

In the United States, pancreatic transplantations have increased from 79 in 1988 to 1221 in 1998. Vascularized pancreatic allograft allows for euglycemia and an insulin-independent state in almost all recipients. One-year graft and patient survival is 69% and 88%, respectively. Simultaneous kidney/pancreas transplantation (SKP) is the most common procedure performed. This procedure is performed in patients with end-stage renal disease resulting from the effects of diabetes. Pancreas transplantation in these patients protects the newly transplanted kidney from recurrent diabetic complications. Pancreas-after-kidney transplantation (PAK) is performed for type 1 diabetics who have had previous kidney transplantation or in patients who have a history of graft pancreatectomy following an SKP procedure. Pancreas transplantation alone (PTA) is indicated for patients with severe metabolic disability, severe autonomic dysfunction, and those who have a creatinine clearance of greater than 30 mL/min. PTA aims to improve quality of life and prevent or delay the onset of frank renal failure and other complications of diabetes.

SUGGESTED READING

Cefalu WT, Skyler JS, Kourides IA, et al. Inhaled human insulin treatment in patients with type 2 diabetes mellitus. *Ann Intern Med.* 2001;134:203-207.

Edelman SV, Henry RR. Insulin therapy for normalizing the glycosylated hemoglobin in type II diabetes: applications, benefits and risks. *Diabetes Review.* 1994;3:308-334.

Mudaliar S, Edelman SV. Insulin therapy in type 2 diabetes. *Endocrinol Metab Clin North Am.* 2001;30:935-982.

Owens DR, Coates PA, Luzio SD, Tinbergen JP, Kurzhals R. Pharmacokinetics of 125I-labeled insulin glargine (HOE 901) in healthy men: comparison with NPH insulin and the influence of different subcutaneous injection sites. *Diabetes Care.* 2000;23:813-819.

Upcoming diabetes medications. In: *Diabetes Monitor.* Independence, Mo: Midwest Diabetes Care Center; April, 1996.

Treatment Algorithm

The primary treatment goals of managing type 2 diabetes are to:

- Eliminate symptoms of hyperglycemia
- Achieve and maintain normal or near-normal metabolic and biochemical parameters (both fasting and postprandial blood glucose levels, glycated hemoglobin [Table 9.1], low-density lipoprotein [LDL] and high-density lipoprotein [HDL] cholesterol, and fasting triglycerides)
- Achieve normal blood pressure and address procoagulant state
- Reduce insulin resistance and its adverse metabolic consequences
- Assist the patient in achieving and maintaining a reasonable body weight
- Prevent or delay the development and progression of microvascular and macrovascular complications.

Therapeutic efforts to achieve these goals involve using a variety of treatment modalities:

- Dietary modifications
- Regular physical activity
- Aspirin therapy
- Oral antidiabetic agents
- Insulin injections.

An individualized approach is recommended based on:

- Patient age
- The presence of coexisting illnesses and/or diabetes-related complications
- Lifestyle, including:

TABLE 9.1 — GLYCEMIC CONTROL FOR PEOPLE WITH DIABETES*

	Normal	Goal	Additional Action Suggested
Whole blood values			
Average preprandial glucose[†]	<100 mg/dL	80-120 mg/dL	<80 mg/dL or >140 mg/dL
Average bedtime glucose[†]	<110 mg/dL	100-140 mg/dL	<100 mg/dL or >160 mg/dL
Plasma values			
Average preprandial glucose[‡]	<110 mg/dL	90-130 mg/dL	<90 mg/dL / >150 mg/dL
Average bedtime glucose[‡]	<120 mg/dL	110-150 mg/dL	<110 mg/dL / >180 mg/dL
HbA$_{1C}$	<6%	<7%	>8%

* The values shown in this table are by necessity generalized to the entire population of individuals with diabetes. Patients with comorbid diseases, the very young and older adults, and others with unusual conditions or circumstances may warrant different treatment goals. These values are for nonpregnant adults. Additional action suggested depends on individual patient circumstances. Such actions may include enhanced diabetes self-management education, comanagement with a diabetes team, referral to an endocrinologist, change in pharmacological therapy, initiation of or increase in self monitoring of blood glucose, or more frequent contact with the patient. HbA$_{1C}$ is referenced to a nondiabetic range of 4.0% to 6.0% (mean 5.0%, SD 0.5%).

† Measurement of capillary blood glucose.

‡ Values calibrated to plasma glucose.

- Attitudes
- Habits
- Cultural/ethnic status
- Financial considerations
- Ability to learn and follow self-management skills
- Level of patient motivation.

The cornerstone of effective diabetes management is maintaining good glycemic control. Compelling evidence indicates that long-term glycemic control can prevent or delay the microvascular complications of diabetes. The Diabetes Control and Complications Trial (DCCT) and the United Kingdom Prospective Diabetes Study (UKPDS) demonstrated definitively the value of improved glycemic therapy of patients with type 1 and type 2 diabetes in delaying the onset and slowing the progression of retinopathy, nephropathy, and neuropathy. The benefits of reducing glycemia are seen in both type 1 and type 2 diabetes.

The American Diabetes Association (ADA) now recommends establishing a management goal of achieving the best possible blood glucose control in patients with type 2 diabetes. Treatment methods for managing type 2 diabetes should focus on:
- Dietary modifications
- Exercise
- Weight control
- Supplemental oral hypoglycemic agents and/or insulin as needed.

The following algorithm (Figure 9.1) provides a general guideline for making decisions regarding the various types of pharmacologic therapy.

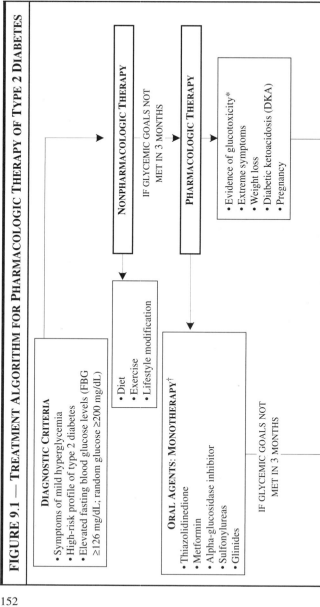

FIGURE 9.1 — TREATMENT ALGORITHM FOR PHARMACOLOGIC THERAPY OF TYPE 2 DIABETES

DIAGNOSTIC CRITERIA
- Symptoms of mild hyperglycemia
- High-risk profile of type 2 diabetes
- Elevated fasting blood glucose levels (FBG ≥126 mg/dL; random glucose ≥200 mg/dL)

NONPHARMACOLOGIC THERAPY

IF GLYCEMIC GOALS NOT MET IN 3 MONTHS

- Diet
- Exercise
- Lifestyle modification

PHARMACOLOGIC THERAPY

- Evidence of glucotoxicity*
- Extreme symptoms
- Weight loss
- Diabetic ketoacidosis (DKA)
- Pregnancy

ORAL AGENTS: MONOTHERAPY†
- Thiazolidinedione
- Metformin
- Alpha-glucosidase inhibitor
- Sulfonylureas
- Glinides

IF GLYCEMIC GOALS NOT MET IN 3 MONTHS

ORAL AGENTS: COMBINED THERAPY†

- Thiazolidinedione + metformin
- Thiazolidinedione + sulfonylurea or glinides
- Alpha-glucosidase inhibitor + sulfonylurea or glinides
- Metformin + sulfonylurea or glinides
- Any combination is feasible, including drugs in triple combination‡

OR§

COMBINED: INSULIN + ORAL AGENT†

- Single bedtime intermediate- or long-acting insulin (adjusted to reduce FBG to <120 mg/dL consistently) plus daytime oral agent(s)

IF DAYTIME GLYCEMIA NOT ACHIEVED IN 3 MONTHS, DISCONTINUE OR ADD/CHANGE ORAL AGENT

INSULIN ALONE¶

- Split-mixed regimen: intermediate- and fast-acting (70/30, 75/25), prebreakfast and predinner
- Multiple injections (3 or more) ± long-acting insulin
- Continuous subcutaneous insulin infusion (CSII)

IF HYPERGLYCEMIA INADEQUATELY CONTROLLED (HbA₁C >8.0%) AND USING >30-75 U/DAY INSULIN

ADD THIAZOLIDINEDIONE OR METFORMIN OR ALPHA-GLUCOSIDASE INHIBITOR, EXCEPT DKA AND PREGNANCY

---

* Insulin use may be temporary to reduce glucotoxicity; patient then may respond to sulfonylureas and other oral agents, alone or in combination.

† Choice of therapy depends on individual patient characteristics.

‡ Many combinations not yet FDA-approved indication.

§ Patient selection for combination therapy (see *Combination Therapy* in Chapter 8, *Insulin Therapy*).

¶ Choice of insulin regimen based on individual assessment.

9

SUGGESTED READING

American Diabetes Association. Clinical practice recommendations 1995. Standards of medical care for patients with diabetes mellitus. *Diabetes Care*. 1995;18(suppl 1):8-15.

American Diabetes Association. *Medical Management of Non–insulin-dependent (Type II) Diabetes*, 3rd ed. Alexandria, Va: American Diabetes Association; 1994:22-39.

American Diabetes Association. Position statement. Standards of medical care for patients with diabetes mellitus. *Diabetes Care*. 1991;14:10-13.

Mudaliar S, Henry RR. Combination therapy for type 2 diabetes. *Endocrinol Pract*. 1999;5:208-219.

Ohkubo Y, Kishikawa H, Araki E, et al. Intensive insulin therapy prevents the progression of diabetic microvascular complications in Japanese patients with non–insulin-dependent diabetes mellitus: a randomized prospective 6-year study. *Diabetes Res Clin Pract*. 1995;28:103-117.

United Kingdom Prospective Diabetes Study (UKPDS) Group. Intensive blood-glucose control with sulphonylureas or insulin compared with conventional treatment and risk complications in patients with type 2 diabetes (UKPDS 33). *Lancet*. 1998;352:837-853.

10 Assessment of the Treatment Regimen

Certain key clinical and metabolic parameters should be monitored during office visits:

- To assess glycemic control:
  - Glycosylated hemoglobin level
  - Plasma glucose values
- To assess cardiovascular risk:
  - Lipoprotein analysis
  - Blood pressure
  - Body weight
- To assess for evidence of diabetic complications
  - Kidney test
  - Dilated eye examination
  - Foot examination.

The metabolic goals for these parameters are shown in Table 10.1.

Glycemic control is assessed during office visits with determinations of plasma glucose levels and assays for glycated hemoglobin. Patients can evaluate the effects of their treatment regimen on a day-to-day basis between office visits by using self-monitoring of blood glucose (SMBG) at home. A combination of physician and patient assessment methods is used to obtain the most accurate information about the degree of metabolic control.

TABLE 10.1 — METABOLIC GOALS OF EFFECTIVE MANAGEMENT

- Glycosylated hemoglobin:
  - Within 1 percentage point above the upper range of normal (<7%)
  - Within 3 SD from the mean
- Fasting plasma glucose level between 80 mg/dL and 120 mg/dL
- Two-hour postprandial plasma glucose level <160 mg/dL
- Systolic/diastolic blood pressure <130/85 mmHg if no evidence of proteinuria (<120/80 mmHg with evidence of proteinuria)
- Approach or maintain ideal body weight
- Lipoprotein goals:
  - Triglyceride level <150 mg/dL
  - HDL cholesterol level >45 mg/dL (>55 in women)
  - LDL cholesterol level <100 mg/dL

Measuring Plasma Glucose Concentrations

Day-to-day glycemic control is reflected in measurements of plasma glucose concentrations. However, because this measurement is an isolated finding at a single point in time, it may not represent a patient's usual metabolic state. Some limitations of plasma glucose measurements are:

- It is difficult to know the meaning of a single random or fasting plasma glucose determination.
- Random determinations may reflect peak, trough, or values in-between because of the wide daily variations in glucose levels.
- The stress of an office visit may result in higher than usual glucose values.

- Some patients may become atypically adherent to their treatment regimen or use extra insulin before an office visit, resulting in an uncharacteristically low glucose level.
- The presence of an intercurrent illness at the time of an office visit can alter blood glucose levels.

Home glucose monitoring data are appropriate for assessing glycemic control and making changes in the therapeutic regimen of patients being treated with diet, oral agents, and insulin therapy. Inaccurate or suspicious results would be revealed by a glycated hemoglobin assay, which reflects the level of glucose control for the preceding 2 to 3 months. Because a single plasma glucose measurement does not provide an adequate assessment of any type of therapy, other corroborating data are needed such as symptoms of hypoglycemia or uncontrolled diabetes, a glycated hemoglobin value, and repeated plasma glucose measurements.

The timing of plasma glucose measurements has an impact on the significance of the findings:
- A postprandial sample obtained 1 to 2 hours after a patient has eaten is the most sensitive measurement because glucose levels are the highest during this time; total carbohydrate content of the meal will be reflected in this glucose value.
- A preprandial or fasting plasma glucose level reflects how efficiently carbohydrates from a meal have been cleared from the plasma.

Measuring Glycated Hemoglobin

Assays of HbA_1, HbA_{1C}, and glycated hemoglobin are used extensively to provide an accurate time-integrated measure of average glycemic control over the previous 2 to 3 months and to correlate plasma glucose measurements and patients' SMBG results. Because these assays do not reflect the glucose level at the time a blood sample is tested, measurements of glycated hemoglobin are not useful for making day-to-day adjustments in the treatment regimen.

Glycation refers to a carbohydrate-protein linkage. This irreversible process occurs as glucose in the plasma attaches itself to the hemoglobin component of red blood cells. Because the lifespan of red blood cells is 120 days, glycated hemoglobin assays reflect average blood glucose concentration over that time.

The amount of circulating glucose concentration to which the red cell is exposed influences the amount of glycated hemoglobin. Therefore, the hyperglycemia of diabetes causes an increase in the percentage of glycated hemoglobin in patients with diabetes; HbA_{1C} shows the greatest change, whereas the remaining glycated hemoglobins are relatively stable.

Levels of HbA_{1C} and HbA_1 correlate best with the degree of diabetic control obtained several months earlier. Regardless of which assay is used, however, certain conditions can interfere with obtaining accurate results:

- False low concentrations are likely in the presence of conditions that decrease the life of the red blood cell, such as:
  - Hemolytic anemia
  - Bleeding
  - Sickle cell trait
- False high concentrations are likely in the presence of conditions that increase the lifespan of the red blood cell, eg, patients without a spleen. Other conditions that produce falsely elevated glycated hemoglobins include:
  - Uremia
  - High concentrations of fetal hemoglobin

- High aspirin doses (>10 g/day)
- High concentrations of ethanol.

Regular monitoring of glycated hemoglobin (eg, every 3 to 6 months) is essential for all patients with diabetes regardless of their type of therapy. On a daily basis, patients typically measure capillary blood glucose levels before meals, postprandially, and at bedtime, particularly with intensive insulin regimens in which near-normal glycemia is being actively pursued. Even when preprandial levels seem satisfactory, patients' glycated hemoglobin results often are higher than expected. This finding would not have been evident through glucose measurements alone, and the need for further efforts to control blood glucose would not have been apparent without obtaining a glycated hemoglobin measurement. Home glycosylated hemoglobin testing is now available (Becton-Dickinson). The patient applies a drop of blood to a reagent card, which is mailed into a central laboratory. The results are then mailed back to the patient.

A disposable test kit for glycosylated HbA_{1c} is now available for home testing by patients with diabetes (Metrika).

10

Measuring Other Glycated Proteins

Enhanced glycation of other proteins occurs in diabetes and has been proposed as another method of assessing average glucose control. Because of the shorter half-life of serum proteins (17 to 20 days) compared with hemoglobin (56 days), measurement of serum fructosamine reflect a shorter period of average glucose control (2 to 3 weeks). Traditionally, fructosamine measurements are particularly useful for following patients with gestational diabetes. Until recently, the clinical utility of fructosamine testing was limited because patients are not normally seen every 2 to 3 weeks. A home fructosamine/glucose meter is now available (The InCharge, LXN Corporation) that measures both glucose and fructosamine with a hand-held device using a drop of blood. Since the results are immediate and the patient can do this test easily at home, the fructosamine value takes on greater importance. Patients do not need venopuncture and there is no delay in getting the results and interpretation from the doctor's office. Although the units are different, they are closely correlated with the HbA_{1C}, ie, a HbA_{1C} of 8% equals a fructosamine value of 325 µmol/L (Figure 10.1).

New devices that are available or soon to be released will have the capabilities of measuring serum ketones, lipoproteins, microalbumin, and other important clinical measurements that traditionally could only be obtained by venupuncture or urine collection and measured in a laboratory.

Self-Monitoring of Blood Glucose

This method of self-evaluation using capillary blood samples has become one of the most important tools for monitoring and improving glycemic control and making adjustments in the diabetes therapeutic regimen. SMBG is a relatively painless procedure that involves pricking the fingertip with a lancet to obtain a drop of blood that is placed on a test strip. Reagents on the test strip contain an enzyme that causes glucose to react with a dye to produce a color change. The color intensity is proportional to the amount of glucose present. The test strip is placed in a small, hand-held meter that quantifies the glucose concentration using reflectance spectrometry. Some test strips can be read visually; other systems measure the electrical current produced by the glucose oxidation reaction to quantify the glucose concentration. Results

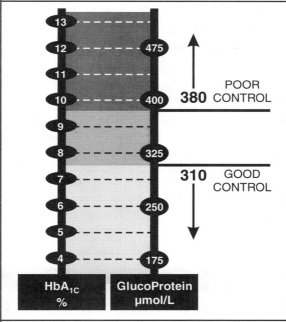

FIGURE 10.1 — COOPERATIVE RELATIONSHIP BETWEEN FRUCTOSAMINE AND HbA$_{1C}$ VALUES

HbA$_{1C}$ %	GlucoProtein µmol/L
13	
12	475
11	
10	400
9	
8	325
7	
6	250
5	
4	175

POOR CONTROL **380**

GOOD CONTROL **310**

This figure shows the equivalent relationship between fructosamine (glucoprotein) values, which reflect the prior 2 to 3 *weeks* of control, compared with the more commonly used HbA$_{1C}$ values, which reflect the prior 2 to 3 *months* of control.

obtained by SMBG tend to have good agreement with plasma glucose concentrations obtained by clinical laboratory procedures if done properly. Patient technique tends to be the source of most discrepancies. Typically, plasma venous glucose measurements are within 15% of the results of whole blood capillary glucose determinations.

Self-monitoring of blood glucose is not a goal in itself but rather a means of achieving the goal of normal or near-normal glycemic control. It should be considered an important part of a comprehensive treatment regimen that includes:

- Diabetes education
- Counseling
- Management by a multidisciplinary team of health care providers.

Goals of treatment and thus the reason for performing SMBG must be clearly defined for the patient. Patients must be motivated and capable of learning the proper techniques of SMBG and committed to applying the results to modify their treatment. Health care providers must be able to discuss SMBG results in a nonderogatory, helpful way that provides encouragement through open, honest communication and an atmosphere of support.

Reasons for Performing SMBG

The following reasons for performing SMBG have been outlined in a consensus statement by the American Diabetes Association:

1. *To achieve or maintain a specific level of glycemic control* — As evidenced by results of the Diabetes Control and Complications Trial (DCCT) and United Kingdom Prospective Diabetes Study (UKPDS), intensive therapy that is closely monitored using SMBG can help patients achieve near-normoglycemia and delay the onset and slow the progression of diabetic complications in type 1 diabetes and type 2 diabetes. Therefore, SMBG at least four times daily is essential for evaluating and adjusting insulin doses in patients on intensive insulin regimens and, with lesser fre-

quency, for patients on less complex insulin or combination regimens or those using oral agents and diet, directed toward achieving near-normoglycemia.

2. *To prevent and detect hypoglycemia* — Hypoglycemia is a major complication of treatment regimens, particularly those involving intensive application of pharmacologic therapy to achieve near-normoglycemia. The elderly are particularly susceptible to hypoglycemia, and certain oral antidiabetic agents such as the sulfonylureas can produce hypoglycemia. Therefore, appropriately timed SMBG is the only way to detect asymptomatic hypoglycemia so that appropriate action (adjusting insulin/oral agents, modifying diet/exercise) can be taken to prevent it from becoming severe.

3. *To avoid severe hyperglycemia* — Illness and certain drugs that alter insulin secretion (eg, phenytoin, thiazide diuretics) or insulin action (eg, prednisone) can increase the risk of severe hyperglycemia and/or ketoacidosis. SMBG should be initiated or used more frequently in all of these situations to detect hyperglycemia before it becomes severe. In addition, patients on insulin therapy can use SMBG data to adjust their insulin doses to avoid severe hyperglycemia.

4. *To adjust care in response to lifestyle changes in patients on pharmacologic therapy* — Glucose levels change in response to variations in diet, exercise, and stressful situations. SMBG can help identify patterns of response to planned exercise and daily activity and help modify pharmacologic therapy during times of increased or decreased caloric consumption.

10

Advantages and Disadvantages of SMBG

Self-monitoring of blood glucose enables the patient to be involved in self-management and provides immediate feedback regarding the impact of diet, exercise, and pharmacologic therapy on blood glucose levels. Patients who are educated about SMBG, how to use the results, and how to make self adjustments of insulin doses using algorithms (for insulin-requiring type 2 patients and type 1 patients) can achieve better daily glycemic control and have a better sense of self-control and participation in their own care. SMBG also provides worthwhile feedback that the physician and other members of the diabetes health care team can incorporate into ongoing evaluation of the treatment regimen. However, health care professionals need to make a point of requesting and reviewing a patient's SMBG data to provide helpful guidance and encouragement.

Advantages of SMBG include:
- Accurate, immediate results for detecting hypoglycemia and hyperglycemia
- Day-to-day assessment of glycemic control
- Follow-up information after changes in treatment to enhance accurate adjustments in pharmacologic therapy
- Enhanced patient independence, self-confidence, and participation in their treatment
- Storage of test results.

Disadvantages of SMBG include:
- Discomfort of lancing the finger to obtain blood (many meters today have alternate site testing)
- Complexity of some testing procedures, requiring mental acuity and dexterity

- Potential malfunction of equipment that could lead to inaccurate results that may affect treatment decisions
- False results because of inaccurate technique that may affect treatment decisions.

SMBG Systems

A combination of factors affect the overall performance of SMBG systems:
- The analytic performance of the meter
- The ability of the user
- The quality of the test strips
- The downloading capacity of home and office computers

Analytic error can range from 4% to 33%; a goal of future SMBG systems is an analytic error of ± 5%. User performance is most affected by the quality and extent of training, which currently is hindered by reimbursement policies for diabetes education. Initial and regular assessments of a patient's SMBG technique is necessary to assure accurate results. Patients need to be advised that test strips can be adversely affected by environmental factors. In addition, cautious use of generic test strips is warranted because of the complex process of calibrating test strips to specific meters.

Examples and features of available blood glucose meters are shown in Tables 10.2 and 10.3. The American Diabetes Association (ADA) Consensus Panel advises periodic comparisons between a patient's SMBG system and a sample obtained simultaneously and measured by a referenced laboratory. Remember that whole blood glucose values are generally 15% lower than plasma values.

TABLE 10.2 — BLOOD GLUCOSE MONITORS: SPECIFICATIONS

Product (Manufacturer)	Weight (oz)	Test Strip Used*	Range (mg/dL)	Test Time	Battery	Warranty
Accu-Chek Active (Roche Diagnostics)	1.56	Accu-Chek Active	10-600	5 sec	(2) CR2023 or equivalent lithium	3 y
Accu-Chek Advantage (Roche Diagnostics)	2.10 w/o batteries	Accu-Chek Advantage or Accu-Chek Comfort Curve	10-600	26 sec	(2) AAA	3 y
Accu-Chek Complete (Roche Diagnostics)	4.4 w/o batteries	Accu-Chek Advantage or Accu-Chek Comfort Curve	10-600	26 sec	(2) AAA	3 y
Accu-Chek Voicemate (Roche Diagnostics)	10.94 w/o batteries	Accu-Chek Comfort Curve	10-600	20 sec	9-volt for the voice synthe-sizer; 3-volt lithium for meter	3 y
Assure (Hypoguard)	5.3	Assure	30-550	35 sec	(1) J-cell (home change)	3 y
Assure II (Hypoguard)	2.2 w/ battery	Assure II	30-550	30 sec	(1) 3-volt lithium	3 y
AtLast (Amira Medical)	3.2	AtLast	40-400	15 sec	Permanent, no replacement required; 2500 tests	3 y or 2500 tests
CheckMate Plus (QuestStar Medical)	1.8 w/ batteries	CheckMate Plus	25-500	15-70 sec	(2) 3-volt lithium	Lifetime

166

	7.0 w/ battery	Duet Glucose Test Strip/ Glucoprotein Test Strip	20-600/ 150-700‡	8-30 sec/4 min	(4) AAA	4 y
Duet† (LXN)	7.0 w/ battery	Duet Glucose Test Strip/ Glucoprotein Test Strip	20-600/ 150-700‡	8-30 sec/4 min	(4) AAA	4 y
ExacTech (Abbott/MediSense)	1.7	ExacTech	40-450	30 sec	Permanent, no replacement required; 4000 tests	4 y
ExacTech RSG (Abbott/MediSense)	1.4	ExacTech RSG	40-450	30 sec	Permanent, no replacement required; 4000 tests	4 y
FreeStyle (TheraSense)	2.1	FreeStyle	20-500	15 sec	(2) AAA (home change)	5 y
Glucometer DEX (Bayer)	2.8	Glucometer DEX	20-600	30 sec	(2) 3-volt lithium (CR-2016)	5 y
Glucometer Elite (Bayer)	1.75	Glucometer Elite	20-600	30 sec	(2) 3-volt lithium	5 y
Glucometer Elite XL (Bayer)	2.1	Glucometer Elite	20-600	30 sec	(2) 3-volt lithium	5 y
Glucometer Encore (Bayer)	3.6	Glucometer Encore	10-600	15 sec	Permanent; 5-y warranty	3 y
InCharge† (LXN)	2.1 w/ battery	In Charge Glucose/ In Charge GlucoProtein	20-600/ 150-700‡	5-20 sec/4 min	3-volt 2032 lithium	3 y
MediSense 2 Card (Abbott)	1.7	MediSense 2 or Precision QID	20-600	20 sec	Permanent, no replacement required; 4000 tests	4 y

Continued

10

Product (Manufacturer)	Weight (oz)	Test Strip Used*	Range (mg/dL)	Test Time	Battery	Warranty
MediSense 2 Pen (Abbott)	1.1	MediSense 2 or Precision QID	20-600	20 sec	Permanent, no replacement required; 4000 tests	4 y
MiniMed CGMS (Medtronic MiniMed)	4.0	None	40-400	Continuously for 72 h	(2) AAA alkaline 1.5-volt	Limited 1 y
One Touch Basic (LifeScan)	4.1	One Touch	0-600	45 sec	(2) AAA (home change)	3 y
One Touch FastTake (LifeScan)	1.6	FastTake	20-600	15 sec	2 silver oxide #357 (1.5-volt; home change)	3 y
One Touch Profile (LifeScan)	4.5	One Touch	0-600	45 sec	(2) AAA (home change)	5 y
One Touch SureStep (LifeScan)	3.8	SureStep	0-500	15-30 sec	(2) AAA alkaline (home change)	3 y
OneTouch Ultra (LifeScan)	1.5	One Touch Ultra	20-600	5 sec	1 replaceable 3-volt (#2032 or equivalent) lithium battery	3 y
Prestige IQ (Home Diagnostics)	<3 w/o battery	Prestige Smart System	25-600	10-50 sec	AAA	5 y
Prestige LX (Home Diagnostics)	4.9	Prestige Smart System	25-600	10-50 sec	6-volt J-cell	5 y

168

Precision Xtra (Abbott/MediSense)	2.76	20-500	20 sec/glucose; 30 sec/ketones	(2) AAA (home change)	4 y
ReliOn (Wal-Mart)	1.5	20-600	20 sec	No replacement required; 4000 tests	4000 tests
Sof-Tact (Abbott/MediSense)	11	30-450	20 sec	1.9 volt	2 y
Supreme II (Hypoguard)	4.7	30-600	50 sec	(1) J-cell (home change)	3 y

*All home meters test whole blood, but some of the newer meters give results in plasma values, the same as you would get from a laboratory test.

† Combination blood glucose monitor and glycated protein test.

‡ Glycated protein range (mmol/L).

Adapted from: *Diabetes Forecast.* 2002;55:75-83.

10

TABLE 10.3 — BLOOD GLUCOSE MONITORS: FEATURES

Product (Manufacturer)	Control Solution	Calibration Method	Features
Accu-Chek Active (Roche Diagnostics)	Yes	Snap-in code key	Five-second test results using small sample size; two-step procedure; meter turns on automatically when strip is inserted; data are downloadable
Accu-Chek Advantage (Roche Diagnostics)	Yes	Snap-in code key	Uses touchable strips with small sample size, capillary action, and large target area; a 100-value memory with time and date has download capability
Accu-Chek Complete (Roche Diagnostics)	Yes	Automatic	Two-step test procedure; collects, stores, and analyzes up to 1000 values; push-button selection provides easy information entry; software available to upload test results to personal computer or healthcare team
Accu-Chek Voicemate (Roche Diagnostics)	Yes	Snap-in code key	For the blind and visually impaired; clear, step-by-step voice guide; touchable strips; easy to use and portable; no cleaning required; Lilly brand insulin identification ensures customer of correct insulin formulation
Assure (Hypoguard)	Yes	Calibrator in each box of strips	Data-management system; biosensor technology; 180-test memory; large touch screen display
Assure II (Hypoguard)	Yes	Calibration chip with each box of test strips	Simple, two-step procedure; small sample size; biosensor technology
AtLast (Amira Medical)	Yes	Calibration chip with each box of test strips	All-in-one meter/lancing system eliminates fingersticks by using less-sensitive areas; easy blood sampling with the flexibility of an adjustable lancet holder with six settings; memory with 14-day average; instructional video included

CheckMate Plus (QuestStar Medical)	Yes	Automatic calibration	Display provides words for guidance; lancing device built in; no wiping, blotting, or timing; automatic hematocrit and temperature correction and sample volume check; stores up to 255 results; average glucose reading; clock with four alarms; data port allows downloading to PC; prompts in 6 languages; hands-off lancet injection
Duet* (LXN)	N/A	Use code button to match monitor to strip lot	Comes with glucose control solution and both normal and high glycated protein control solution. Dual-function monitor uses Duet (fructosamine) strip for once-a-week testing of overall diabetes control; icons and audible cues guide testing; monitor automatically recognizes correct strip; memory holds 150 glucose tests and 50 glucoprotein tests saved by time and date; data port for downloading; video upon request
ExacTech (Abbott/MediSense)	Yes	Calibrator in each box of strips	Credit-card size; simple three-step testing procedure; biosensor technology; no cleaning, wiping, or timing; last reading recall and calibration code
ExacTech RSG (Abbott/MediSense)	Yes	Automatic calibration	Requires no calibration or coding; simple three-step testing procedure; biosensor technology; no cleaning, wiping, or timing; last reading recall and calibration code
FreeStyle (TheraSense)	Yes	Built-in button	Virtually painless off-finger testing with small sample (0.3 microliters); unaffected by oxygen, uric acid, aspirin, and by hematocrit from 0% to 60% (those who are anemic or on dialysis will get accurate readings); sample pulled into strip which automatically turns meter on; sample can be retaken using the same sampling area for up to 60 seconds; confirmation beep to let you know the strip is full; 250-test memory with 14-day average
Glucometer DEX (Bayer)	Yes, 3 levels	Automatic calibration	Cartridge-based monitor eliminates individual strip handling; performs 10 tests without reloading; cartridge automatically calibrates monitor for 10 tests; electronic functions automatically validated; sensor actively draws just the amount of blood it needs; advanced data management; download memory for PC tracking; monitor stores up to 100 results with time, date, and averages

Continued

10

Product (Manufacturer)	Control Solution	Calibration Method	Features
Glucometer Elite (Bayer)	Yes	Strip calibration	Turns on automatically when test strip is inserted; 20-test memory and 3-minute automatic shutoff; includes lancing device, 10 test strips, carrying case, control solution, and log book; instructional video available on request
Glucometer Elite XL (Bayer)	Yes	Strip calibration	Turns on when test strip is inserted; 120-test memory with date, time, and 14-day average and 3-minute automatic shutoff; kit includes blood lancing device and lancets, 10 test strips, carrying case, control solution, and log book; video tape available on request
Glucometer Encore (Bayer)	Yes	Single-button calibration by lot of test strips	Automatic shutoff in 3 minutes; stores up to 10 results; includes carrying case, control solution; 10 test strips, and lancets; Spanish instructions available
InCharge* (LXN)	N/A	Use code button to match monitor to strip lot	Dual-function monitor; glucoprotein (fructosamine) test; memory holds 200 glucose tests and 50 glucoprotein tests saved by time and date
MediSense 2 Card (Abbott)	Yes	Calibrator in each box of strips	Provides all the same features as the MediSense 2 Pen Sensor; credit card size; extra large display window; uses same sensor test strips
MediSense 2 Pen (Abbott)	Yes	Calibrator in each box of strips	Biosensor technology; automatic start with hands-off testing; no cleaning, wiping, blotting; timing; pen-size; extended memory; individually wrapped strips
MiniMed CGMS (Medtronic MiniMed)	No	Daily fingersticks	Glucose sensor may be used for up to 3 days; glucose values (up to 864) are collected and stored; glucose sensor sends a continuous signal to the monitor which samples those signals every 10 seconds and stores an average glucose value every 5 minutes; monitor allows for entry of information by patient; monitors are worn as halter devices; system is not affected by sweat, temperature, or drug use; initialization period lasts only 1 hour for every 3 days of patient use; data are retrospective and cannot be assessed by patient; for physician-supervised use, *not* long-term self-care

One Touch Basic (LifeScan)	Yes	Built-in single button	75-test memory with optional display of date and time; simple, 3-step test procedure; large, easy-to-handle test strips; single-button coding
One Touch FastTake (LifeScan)	Yes	Built-in single button	Less painful alternative site testing; small blood sample; 15-second test time; compact; 150-test memory with date and time; capillary-action test strip; near-monitor dosing; 14-day averaging; warning to check ketones at 240 to 600 mg/dL.; data downloading with In Touch software
One Touch Profile (LifeScan)	Yes	Built-in single button	Three-step testing with no timing, wiping, or blotting; large display in English, Spanish, or 17 other languages; notifies when monitor needs cleaning; stores last 250 results with date and time; 14- and 30-day test average; insulin programming; event labeling; some features can be turned on/off
One Touch SureStep (LifeScan)	Yes	Built-in single button	Single-button testing; blue dot confirms sample before test; touchable test strips; off-meter dosing; 10-test memory; large display with universal symbols; 150-test memory with date and time; 14- and 30-day test averaging; data downloading to personal computer
OneTouch Ultra (LifeScan)	Yes	Built-in single button	Less painful alternate-site testing; fast test time; tiny blood sample; easy blood application, including confirmation window; broad operating temperature range (43°F to 111°F); small meter size; 150-test memory with date and time; 14- and 30-day test averaging; no cleaning necessary; data downloading with In Touch Software; warning to check ketones at 240 to 600 mg/dL
Prestige IQ (Home Diagnostics)	Yes	Standard strip	Data management including date and time and 14- and 30-day averaging; easy-to-read large digital display; Internet uploading capabilities; small blood sample; sample confirmation on back of test strip
Prestige LX (Home Diagnostics)	Yes	Standard strip	Three simple steps; one coding button; large easy-to-read display; 365-test memory; confirmation of sufficient blood sample size

Continued

10

173

Product (Manufacturer)	Control Solution	Calibration Method	Features
Precision Xtra (Abbott/MediSense)	Yes	Calibrator in each box of tests strips	Measures both blood glucose and blood ketone levels; fast readings with small amount of blood; not affected by common medications; lighting features; 450-result memory with time and date, and 1-, 2-, and 4-week averaging
ReliOn (Wal-Mart)	No	Calibrator in each box of test strips	No wiping, blotting, timing, or cleaning; biosensor testing platform requiring only a 4-mL blood sample size; wallet-sized carrying case holds lancing device, 10 lancets, and logbook; stores up to 10 results; automatic start
Sof-Tact (Abbott/MediSense)	Yes	Calibrator in each box of test strips	Alternative-site testing (test of forearm and upper arm, obtaining results in 20 seconds); 450-result memory with date and time; 1-, 2-, and 4-week averaging; compatible with Precision Link 2.3 and higher; preload feature allows patients to load meter with test strip and lancet up to 8 hours in advance of testing
Supreme II (Hypoguard)	Yes	Built-in single button	Large display; universal symbols; blood can be applied to test strip inside or outside of monitor; 100-test memory

* Combination blood glucose monitor and glycated protein tests.

Adapted from: *Diabetes Forecast*. 2002;55:75-83.

Who Should Perform SMBG?

Virtually all patients with diabetes should perform SMBG because of the value of this evaluation tool in promoting improved glycemic control and reinforcing adherence to therapy. The frequency of SMBG is dictated by the complexity of the therapeutic regimen. For example, insulin-using type 2 diabetics (particularly those on an intensive regimen) would need to perform more daily SMBG evaluations than patients who are achieving acceptable glycemic control on diet, exercise, and oral agents.

Recommended Frequency of SMBG

The frequency of SMBG varies considerably based on the complexity of the therapeutic regimen and the clinical situation of the individual. In addition to guiding therapy, SMBG also has educational and motivational advantages. For example, intermittent measurements 1 to 2 hours after meals can provide an assessment of glycemic response to various types of foods, thus helping patients learn which foods have the greatest and least impact on blood glucose, as well as how the size of a meal affects glucose levels. SMBG also can help motivate patients (especially obese patients trying to lose weight), because they can observe immediate decreases in their blood glucose levels in response to dietary modifications, exercise, and oral therapy.

Patients who demonstrate consistent, acceptable glucose results may require fewer tests (ie, one to three tests per week). However, testing requirements may increase when metabolic control worsens.

10

Traditionally, SMBG was viewed as not necessary for type 2 patients on diet therapy or oral agents because glucose levels remained relatively stable on these treatment regimens. For these patients, SMBG was recommended only for monitoring short-term adjustments in therapy or for patients at risk of hypoglycemia. Because better glycemic control has been shown to be associated with a greater frequency of SMBG, this evaluation measure now is recommended for all patients, including those not taking insulin. The frequency of testing depends on how stable the patient is. Patients with less than optimal control should monitor their levels more frequently.

Self-monitoring of blood glucose recommendations for patients on diet therapy:

- Prebreakfast – two to three tests per week
- One to 2 hours postdinner – two to three tests per week.

Glucose values from these two important time points, in addition to a glycosylated hemoglobin or fructosamine value every 3 to 6 months, is an efficient way to follow patients on diet and oral agents.

Self-monitoring of blood glucose recommendations for patients using oral agents alone or combination therapy (daytime oral agents, evening insulin):

- Prebreakfast – four to seven tests per week
- Prelunch – two to three tests per week
- Two hours postdinner – two to three tests per week.

Patients in this category generally require one to three tests per day when SMBG values are consistent. Patients can make nonpharmacologic changes in their diabetic regimen depending on the results (Table 10.4).

TABLE 10.4 — TECHNIQUES USED TO ADJUST FOR PREMEAL HYPERGLYCEMIA

Nonpharmacologic
- Increase the time interval between insulin injection and consumption of the meal.
- Consume less than the usual amount of calories.
- Eliminate or replace foods containing refined carbohydrates or that have a high glycemic index, such as fruit exchanges.
- Spread the calories over an extended period of time.
- Exercise lightly after a meal.

Pharmacologic
- Increase the amount of fast-acting insulin via an algorithm.
- Make the appropriate long-term adjustment in preceding insulin dose to prevent hyperglycemia at a particular time if a consistent trend is identified.

Edelman SV, Henry RR. Insulin therapy for normalizing glycosylated hemoglobin in type II diabetes: application, benefits, and risks. *Diabetes Reviews*. 1994;3:310.

SMBG for Patients Who Take Insulin

Self-monitoring of blood glucose is critical for all patients who take exogenous insulin, particularly those on intensive insulin regimens or on combination therapy. The type of insulin regimen used should dictate the frequency of SMBG, with attention to insulin pharmacokinetics and the timing of insulin injections. The best time to evaluate the effectiveness of a dose is at the peak time of action of a particular type of insulin (see Table 8.1).

Frequent SMBG is necessary to fine-tune an insulin regimen to the needs and responses of a given patient. Ideally, SMBG should be performed four to six times per day (before each meal, at bedtime, and occasionally after meals and at 3:00 AM, which is the approximate time of early morning glucose nadir). A more intensive SMBG schedule would be a pre- and 2-hour postprandial measurement and at bedtime, depending on the frequency of insulin doses.

Self-monitoring of blood glucose recommendations for patients on insulin therapy:

- One injection per day – two tests per day, no less than one to three depending on metabolic control.
- Two injections per day – four tests per day (before each meal and at bedtime)
- Intensive regimen (multiple injections, external pumps) – four to seven tests per day.

Results should be recorded in a log book that is brought to each office visit so the physician can evaluate the effectiveness of the insulin regimen and determine the most appropriate insulin dosage adjustments (Figure 10.2). Selected patients should be instructed to apply their SMBG results as the data become available. Making immediate dosage adjustments based on SMBG feedback is evidence of the true benefit of this self-assessment tool. Additionally, most meter logs can be downloaded directly to a personal computer.

When SMBG reveals premeal hyperglycemia, a number of different methods can be used in addition to adjusting the dose of insulin to reduce daily glycemic excursions (Table 10.4).

Applying SMBG Results to Adjust Insulin Doses

Patients can be taught how to analyze and use SMBG data to effectively make adjustments in their insulin doses so that they can maintain and improve glycemic control. Insulin algorithms can be used with SMBG to make appropriate day-to-day changes in insulin dosing and to guide long-term treatment. The insulin algorithm shown in Figure 10.3 is used for patients receiving intensive insulin therapy. Self-adjustment guidelines for patients on a split-mixed regimen are shown in Table 10.5; insulin unit changes are provided by the physician on an individualized basis.

Advances in Glucose Monitoring

Over the past several years, home glucose monitoring (HGM) devices have become smaller, faster, and easier to operate with data analysis capabilities. Computer-generated data analysis can assist the caregiver and the patient in many different areas, including data collection from blood glucose meters, certain insulin pumps, and other new devices. Computer software programs can also create charts and graphs that reveal trends and patterns in blood glucose values for easier evaluation by the patient and the caregiver. There are many software programs that are not only user friendly for the patient, but are easy to read and analyze by the caregiver. Several programs can generate one-page summaries of a person's diabetes monitoring data intended for optimal presentation of information. Information typically provided includes the standard day plot, before and after meals, pie graphs, the preceding 14 days in a combination graph format (where diet, exercise, and medication is shown with blood sugar levels) and a glucose line plot. The goal ranges and usual insulin doses are usually printed on the bottom of the page if applicable for that patient.

■ Advances in Devices for Blood-Letting

The fingerstick devices used to get a drop of blood for testing from the patient have improved with depth adjustable and sharp, thin lancets. There is a meter that has the capability of getting blood from areas other than the fingertips, such as the forearm, for

FIGURE 10.2 — WEEKLY SELF-MONITORING BLOOD GLUCOSE RECORD SHEET

Name _____

Address _____

City _____

State _____ Zip _____

SSI #: _____ - __ - _____

Home PH#: (___) ___ - ____

Work PH#: (___) ___ - ____

Fax #: (___) ___ - ____

Pager #: (___) ___ - ____

INSTRUCTIONS: Record time of day in upper box and glucose readings in lower box.

Day/Date (m/d/y)	AM Breakfast		AM INSULIN	Noon	PM Dinner		PM INSULIN	Comments
	Before	After			Before	After		
SUNDAY __/__/__								
MONDAY __/__/__								
TUESDAY __/__/__								

180

							Weekly Averages
WEDNESDAY __/__/__							
THURSDAY __/__/__							
FRIDAY __/__/__							
SATURDAY __/__/__							

Daily Averages

	SUNDAY	MONDAY	TUESDAY	WEDNESDAY	THURSDAY	FRIDAY	SATURDAY
TIMES OF DAY							
GLUCOSE READINGS							
WEIGHT							

TOTAL UNITS FOR THE WEEK: AM _____ + PM _____ =

10

181

FIGURE 10.3 — ALGORITHM FORM USED FOR PATIENTS ON INTENSIVE INSULIN THERAPY

Name _____ Date _____

Provider _____ Phone _____

Time Between Injection/Meal (min)		Blood Glucose Value (mg/dL)	Breakfast	Lunch	Dinner	Bedtime	Bedtime Snack Size
Humalog	*Regular*						
0	5-15	<80					Large
5	30	81-150					Medium
5-15	30-45	151-200					Small
15-30	45-60	201-250					None
30	60	251-300					None
30+	60+	301-350					None
30+	60+	351-400					None
30+	60+	401-450					None
30+	60+	451+					None

AM long-acting insulin dose _____

PM long-acting insulin dose _____ ☐ Take before dinner ☐ Take at bedtime

As the premeal blood glucose value increases, the amount of regular insulin recommended also increases and is adjusted based on postprandial glucose values. The time between the insulin injection and the meal also should be increased as the premeal blood glucose values increase, thus improving postprandial glucose values. If the patient consistently requires higher regular insulin doses at a particular time (3 consecutive days), appropriate long-term adjustments should be made.

Diabetes Clinic, VA San Diego Healthcare System, San Diego, California.

TABLE 10.5 — PATIENT SELF ADJUSTMENT OF INSULIN DOSAGE, SPLIT-MIXED REGIMEN

High Glucose Values

1. If the prebreakfast blood sugar is greater than 140 mg/dL for 3 days in a row, then increase the evening NPH dosage by _____ units.

2. If the prelunch blood sugar is greater than 150 mg/dL for 3 days in a row, then increase the morning regular insulin dosage by _____ units.

3. If the predinner blood sugar is greater than 150 mg/dL for 3 days in a row, then increase the morning NPH insulin dosage by _____ units.

4. If the bedtime blood sugar is greater than 180 mg/dL for 3 days in a row, then increase the predinner regular insulin dosage by _____ units.

Low Glucose Values

1. If the prebreakfast blood sugar is less than 100 mg/dL for 3 days in a row, then decrease the evening NPH insulin dosage by _____ units.

2. If the prelunch blood sugar is less than 100 mg/dL for 3 days in a row, then decrease the morning regular insulin dosage by _____ units.

3. If the predinner blood sugar is less than 100 mg/dL for 3 days in a row, then decrease the morning NPH insulin dosage by _____ units.

4. If the bedtime blood sugar is less than 100 mg/dL for 3 days in a row, then decrease the predinner regular insulin dosage by _____ units.

General Considerations

1. If more than one change in insulin dosage is needed, adjust the NPH dosage first before making any changes in the regular dosage.

2. Remember not to make changes in the insulin dosage more frequently than every 3 days, and do not hesitate to call me for any questions at (_____)_____-_____.

_____
Physician/Caregiver

Diabetes Clinic, VA San Diego Healthcare System, San Diego, California.

patient comfort and convenience. Other companies have developed blood-letting devices that can be used on the fingertips and other areas with special attachments to the "finger sticker." Laser technology has also been designed to facilitate the blood-letting for these home devices.

■ Advances in Continuous Glucose Monitoring

The development of devices to allow for frequently measured or real-time glucose values has tremendous implications for achieving near normalization of glucose control while avoiding the most serious complication of intensive glucose management, hypoglycemia. Patient and caregiver education on how to react to frequently obtained values is needed to obtain the maximum benefit from this technology.

The GlucoWatch Automatic Glucose Biographer (Cygnus) provides a means to obtain frequent, automatic, and noninvasive glucose measurements—up to three readings per hour for as long as 12 hours after a single blood glucose measurement for calibration. Clinical studies with the GlucoWatch in controlled laboratory and home environments have demonstrated accuracy and precision, similar to currently available invasive home meters. The GlucoWatch extracts glucose through the skin by reverse iontophoresis and measures the extracted sample using an electrochemical biosensor. Iontophoresis is a technique whereby a low-level electric current is passed through the skin between an anode and a cathode. The amount of glucose extracted at the cathode has been previously demonstrated to correlate with blood glucose in diabetic subjects.

The GlucoWatch has an adjustable low and high glucose alert function, as well as a sweating sensor, and can store several thousand data points. In addition, an alarm will go off if the blood glucose values drop more than 30% between any two values to help avoid a severe hypoglycemic reaction.

There are several other companies currently working on totally noninvasive methods to measure glucose, such as infrared technology and implantable sensors, that are durable and accurate. Invasive frequent glucose monitoring systems are also being developed. The currently available Medtronic continuous glucose monitoring system is a pager-size device that can measure a patient's glucose value every 5 minutes for up to 72 hours. The glucose oxidase sensor, which is located inside a small needle, is placed in the subcutaneous tissue and discarded when removed. The patient is blinded to the information, however. When returned to the caregiver after 3 days, the stored data can be analyzed for trends. These devices are currently available from physicians who have purchased the monitoring system. Future generations of this sensor will communicate with an external insulin pump and provide real-time data.

SUGGESTED READING

American Diabetes Association. Clinical practice recommendations 2000. Tests of glycemia in diabetes. *Diabetes Care*. 2000;23(suppl 1):S80-S83.

American Diabetes Association. *Medical Management of Non–insulin-dependent (Type II) Diabetes*, 3rd ed. Alexandria, Va: American Diabetes Association; 1994:52-54.

Diabetes Control and Complications Trial Research Group. The effect of intensive treatment of diabetes on the development and progression of long-term complications in insulin-dependent diabetes mellitus. *N Engl J Med*. 1993;329: 977-986.

Fleming DR. Accuracy of blood glucose monitoring for patients: what it is and how to achieve it. *Diabetes Educ*. 1994;20:495-500.

Greyson J. Quality control in patient self-monitoring of blood glucose. *Diabetes Care*. 1993;16:1306-1308.

Harris MI, Cowie CC, Howie LJ. Self-monitoring of blood glucose by adults with diabetes in the Unites States population. *Diabetes Care*. 1993;16:1116-1123.

Nettles A. User error in blood glucose monitoring. The National Steering Committee for Quality Assurance report. *Diabetes Care*. 1993;16:946-948.

Peragallo-Dittko V, ed. *A Core Curriculum for Diabetes Education*, 2nd ed. Chicago, Ill: American Association of Diabetes Educators; 1993:259-279.

Porte D, Sherwin RS. *Ellenberg & Rifkin's Diabetes Mellitus*. 5th ed. Stamford, Conn: Appleton & Lange; 1997.

United Kingdom Prospective Diabetes Study (UKPDS) Group. Intensive blood-glucose control with sulphonylureas or insulin compared with conventional treatment and risk complications in patients with type 2 diabetes (UKPDS 33). *Lancet*. 1998;352:837-853.

10

11   Acute Complications

Patients with type 2 diabetes are prone to developing acute complications such as:
- Metabolic:
  - Diabetic ketoacidosis (DKA)
  - Hyperosmolar hyperglycemic nonketotic syndrome (HHNS)
  - Hypoglycemia
- Infection (poor wound healing)
- Quality of life:
  - Nocturia
  - Poor sleep
  - Daytime tiredness
  - Tooth and gum disease
  - Cognitive impairment.

The most common acute complications of diabetes are metabolic problems (DKA, HHNS, hypoglycemia) and infection. In addition, the quality of life of patients with chronic and severe hypoglycemia is adversely affected. Characteristic symptoms of tiredness and lethargy can become severe and lead to increased falls in the elderly, decreased school performance in children, and decreased work performance in adults.

Metabolic

■ Diabetic Ketoacidosis

This acute metabolic complication typically results from a profound insulin deficiency (absolute or relative) associated with uncontrolled type 1 diabetes mellitus and less commonly in severely decompensated type 2 diabetes.

Individuals with type 2 diabetes may develop DKA under certain conditions:

- Poor nutrition that contributes to dehydration and catabolism of fat to provide necessary calories
- Severe physiologic stress (eg, infection, myocardial infarction) that leads to increased levels of counterregulatory hormones (eg, epinephrine, cortisol, and glucagon), which stimulate lipolysis, elevate free fatty acids, and stimulate hepatic ketogenesis
- Chronic poor metabolic control that leads to decreased insulin secretion and decreased glucose uptake (glucose toxicity)
- Dehydration that leads to decreased excretion of ketones in urine and a buildup of ketone bodies in the blood.

Key characteristics include:

- Hyperglycemia (300 to 800 mg/dL although usually <600 mg/dL. The glucose concentration is not related to severity of DKA)
- Ketosis: serum ketones usually 10 to 20 mM and acidosis (pH 6.8-7.3, HCO_3 <15 mEq/L)
- Dehydration caused by:
  - Nausea
  - Vomiting
  - Inadequate oral intake
- Electrolyte depletion (eg, potassium, magnesium, etc).

Precipitating factors vary from individual to individual and may include the following (approximately 50% of which are preventable):

- Illness and infection; increased production of glucagon and glucocorticoids by adrenal gland promotes gluconeogenesis; increased production of epinephrine and norepinephrine increases glycogenolysis

- Inadequate insulin dosage due to omission or reduction of doses by patient, physician, or clinic; patients with gastrointestinal (GI) distress often decrease or eliminate their insulin doses thinking that less insulin is needed when food intake is decreased; this practice can be dangerous because GI symptoms are key features of DKA
- Initial manifestation of type 1 diabetes in the elderly misdiagnosed as type 2 diabetes
- Chronic untreated hyperglycemia (glucose toxicity) and hyperinsulinemia.

Pathophysiology of DKA

Diabetic ketoacidosis is a metabolic acidosis caused by a significant insulin deficiency. The following physiologic abnormalities are characteristic of DKA and require prompt correction:
- Chronic hyperglycemia and glucose toxicity
- Acidosis caused by catabolism of fat and the buildup of ketone bodies
- Low blood volume because of dehydration (loss of fluid and electrolytes)
- Hyperosmolality because of renal water loss and water depletion from sweating, nausea, and vomiting; and associated potassium loss.

Symptoms and Signs of DKA

The symptoms and signs of DKA are shown in Table 11.1. These are classic for DKA in type 1 diabetes, although they are not as severe in patients with type 2 diabetes because some insulin secretion is maintained. Polyuria and polydipsia are symptoms of osmotic diuresis secondary to hyperglycemia. Nonspecific symptoms include weakness, lethargy, headache, and myalgia; specific symptoms of DKA are GI and respiratory. The GI symptoms probably are related to the ketosis and/or acidosis. The chief respiratory com-

TABLE 11.1 — Symptoms and Signs of Classic Diabetic Ketoacidosis

Symptoms of DKA
- Nausea
- Vomiting
- Abdominal pain
- Dyspnea
- Myalgia
- Headache
- Anorexia
- Characteristic symptoms of hyperglycemia

Signs of DKA
- Hypothermia
- Hyperpnea (Kussmaul's respiration)
- Acetone breath
- Dehydration (intravascular volume depletion, hypotension)
- Hyporeflexia
- Acute abdomen (tenderness to palpation, muscle guarding, diminished bowel sounds)
- Stupor (mild to frank coma)
- Hypotonia
- Uncoordinated ocular movements

Abbreviations: DKA, diabetic ketoacidosis.

Davidson MB. *Diabetes Mellitus: Diagnosis and Treatment*, 3rd ed. New York, NY: Churchill Livingstone; 1991.

plaint of dyspnea actually is an inability to catch one's breath. This type of hyperventilation unrelated to exertion is the ventilatory response to metabolic acidosis termed Kussmaul's respiration.

Because the signs are not specific to DKA, physicians should be alert to a constellation of evidence that points to the possibility of DKA.

Because other diseases and conditions may mimic DKA and precipitate and/or coexist with DKA, the following differential diagnoses (and representative DKA symptoms) should be considered:

- Cerebrovascular accident (altered mental status)
- Brainstem hemorrhage (hyperventilation, glucosuria)
- Hypoglycemia (altered mental status, tachycardia)
- Metabolic acidosis (hyperventilation, anion gap acidosis):
  - Uremia
  - Salicylates
  - Methanol
  - Ethylene glycol
- Gastroenteritis (nausea, vomiting, abdominal pain)
- Pneumonia (hyperventilation).

Laboratory Evaluation

Initial laboratory values are shown in Table 11.2.

Treatment

Although aggressive therapy is not usually necessary in type 2 diabetes, the following treatment strategies are for severe cases and for true type 1 diabetes misdiagnosed as type 2 diabetes because of the patient's age at presentation. The goals of treatment are to:

- Correct fluid and electrolyte disturbances
- Correct acidosis and ketogenesis
- Restore and maintain normal glucose metabolism.

11

The cornerstones of DKA therapy are administering fluids and insulin immediately. Potassium and phosphate replacement, and bicarbonate therapy also may be necessary for certain patients, depending on the severity of the DKA. This is rarely the case in patients with type 2 diabetes. The following treatment guidelines provide an overview for managing DKA. It is not unusual that patients with type 2 diabetes can be treated adequately in a general hospital ward and not in an intensive care unit.

TABLE 11.2 — INITIAL LABORATORY VALUES FOR PATIENTS EXPERIENCING DIABETIC KETOACIDOSIS

Test	Result	Remarks
Glucose	300-800 mg/dL	Concentrations not related to severity of DKA
Ketone bodies	Strong at least in undiluted plasma	Measures only acetoacetate, not β-hydroxybutyrate
[HCO$_3$]	0-15 mEq/L	Concentrations related to severity of DKA
pH	6.8-7.3	Concentrations related to severity of DKA
[K]	Low, normal, or high	Total body depletion; heart responsive to extracellular concentration
Phosphate	Usually normal or slightly elevated; occasionally slightly low	Associated with phosphaturia; marked decrease with treatment in levels of both serum and urine phosphates
Creatine/BUN	Usually mildly increased	May be prerenal; spurious increases in creatinine by acetoacetate in some automated methods

WBC count	Usually increased	Possibility of leukemoid reaction (even in absence of infection)
Amylase	Often increased	Predominant form of salivary gland origin
Hemoglobin, hematocrit, total protein	Often increased	Secondary to contracted plasma volume
AST, ALT, LDH	Can be mildly elevated	Spurious increases in transaminases due to acetoacetate interference in older colorimetric methods

Abbreviations: DKA, diabetic keotacidosis; HCO$_3$, concentration of bicarbonate; K, concentration of potassium; BUN, blood urea nitrogen; WBC, white blood cell (count); AST, aspartate aminotransferase; ALT, alanine aminotransferase; LDH, lactic dehydrogenase.

Reprinted with permission from Davidson MB. *Diabetes Mellitus: Diagnosis and Treatment*, 3rd ed. New York, NY: Churchill Livingstone; 1991:183.

Fluid and Electrolyte Replacement

- Based on the degree of dehydration and the patient's cardiovascular status.
- Also plays a critical role in lowering glucose concentrations; hyperglycemia will continue despite appropriate insulin therapy if hydration is not adequate.
- Oral hydration with a sodium-containing fluid is appropriate for a patient with mild DKA who is not vomiting.
- Most adults require IV fluid administration with normal (0.9%) or half-normal (0.45%) saline (normal saline should be used when intravascular volume depletion is extreme and half-normal saline when plasma volume contraction is more moderate).
- One liter of fluid should be given per hour for the first 2 hours; the rate can be decreased to 500 mL per hour when signs of intravascular volume depletion have subsided.
- IV fluids are continued until intravascular volume has been fully restored, as indicated by normal filling of neck veins or when the patient can tolerate fluids.

Insulin Therapy

- Most patients with type 2 diabetes can be treated successfully with frequent (every 2 to 3 hours) injections of Humalog or Novolog insulin subcutaneously (5 to 15 units).
- A low dose of regular insulin can be administered via IV infusion at a rate of approximately 5 units per hour.
- If a 10% decrease in glucose concentration from the initial level is not observed after 2 hours, the infusion rate should be doubled to 10 units per hour.

- The insulin infusion can be discontinued and intermediate-acting NPH insulin can be started when HCO_3 is >15 mEq/L and the patient can drink and eat light foods.
- The major mistake with severe DKA is premature discontinuation of aggressive fluid and insulin therapy. Ketogenesis must be curtailed and requires insulin therapy. Serum glucose levels are not reflective of ketone body generation.

Potassium Replacement

- Not usually necessary in patients with type 2 diabetes
- May be necessary after fluid and insulin therapy have been started because all modes of therapy reduce the serum [K].
- The goal is to maintain the serum [K] within the normal range.
- An ECG should be done as soon as possible. Potassium replacement is withheld if the patient is anuric or if the T waves are abnormally tall and peaked or have a high-normal configuration. If the T waves are normal, 20 mEq of potassium (with appropriate anion) is added to the first liter of replacement fluid. Low or flat T waves require the addition of 40 mEq of potassium.
- An ECG should be taken every 1 to 2 hours to evaluate treatment and adjust the potassium replacement regimen. Patients who are able to eat can receive potassium orally via food intake or potassium supplementation (12 to 15 mEq three times daily with meals).

Phosphate Replacement

- Phosphate levels should be measured initially; some physicians use potassium phosphate for replacement if PO_4 is in the low or low-normal range.

Bicarbonate Therapy

- Not necessary for most patients but may be considered under certain circumstances, such as for patients with life-threatening hyperkalemia, lactic acidosis, or severe acidosis (pH <7.0) with shock that does not respond to fluid replacement.
- When necessary, bicarbonate should be added to 0.45% saline and infused slowly over at least 1 hour; it should never be given in an IV bolus because of the risk of death secondary to hypokalemia.

Glucose concentrations should be decreased by about 75 to 100 mg/dL/h with low-dose insulin infusion, reaching levels of 200 to 300 mg/dL within 4 to 5 hours. Dextrose generally is added to the infusion at this point in therapy to avoid hypoglycemia from continued insulin administration, which still is necessary to treat ketosis and acidosis. Approximately 12 to 24 hours of treatment is necessary to reverse ketosis for most patients; some patients may have ketone bodies for several days.

■ Hyperosmolar Hyperglycemic Nonketotic Syndrome

This acute metabolic complication is a life-threatening crisis with a high mortality rate that usually is seen in:

- Elderly patients with type 2 diabetes (particularly those in nursing homes without access to free water)
- People with undiagnosed diabetes
- Those with diabetes that is diagnosed after a long period of uncontrolled hyperglycemia.

Pathophysiology of HHNS

Hyperosmolar hyperglycemic nonketotic syndrome has four key clinical features:

- Severe hyperglycemia—blood glucose usually >600 mg/dL (>33.3 mM) and generally 1000 mg/dL to 2000 mg/dL (55.5 mM to 111.1 mM)
- Absence of or slight ketosis
- Plasma or serum hyperosmolality (>340 mOsm)
- Profound dehydration.

In clinical practice, patients often are seen who have these characteristics but also have mild ketosis and acidosis. Although HHNS and DKA represent opposite ends of a continuum, many patients have some aspects of each syndrome. The two conditions have some similarity in pathophysiology, clinical signs and symptoms, and treatments, with certain important exceptions.

Symptoms and Signs of HHNS

Patients typically develop excessive thirst, confusion, and physical signs of severe dehydration. A comparison of the key features of HHNS and DKA is shown in Table 11.3; several important differences exist in the symptoms and signs:

- GI symptoms usually are milder in HHNS than in DKA in the absence of ketosis and acidosis. Because of a lack of severe GI problems (which prompted patients with DKA to seek medical attention within 1 to 2 days), patients with HHNS may tolerate polyuria and polydipsia for weeks and consequently lose significant quantities of fluids and electrolytes before seeking help. Average fluid loss in HHNS is 9 L vs 6.5 L in DKA.
- Kussmaul's respiration is rarely observed because of a lack of severe acidosis.

TABLE 11.3 — DIABETIC KETOACIDOSIS AND HYPERGLYCEMIC HYPEROSMOLAR NONKETOTIC SYNDROME: COMPARISON OF SOME SALIENT FEATURES

Feature	Conditions	
	DKA	HHNS
Age of patients	Usually <40 years	Usually >60 years
Duration of symptoms	Usually <2 days	Usually >5 days
Glucose level	Usually <600 mg/dL (<33.3 mmol/L)	Usually >800 mg/dL (>44.4 mmol/L)
Sodium concentration	More likely to be normal, or low	More likely to be normal or high
Potassium concentration	High, normal or low	High, normal, or low
Bicarbonate concentration	Low	Normal
Ketone bodies	At least 4+ in 1:1 dilution	<2+ in 1:1 dilution
pH	Low	Low
Serum osmolality	Usually <350 mOsm/kg (<350 mmol/kg)	Usually >350 mOsm/kg (>350 mmol/kg)

Cerebral edema	Often subclinical; occasionally clinical	Subclinical has not been evaluated; rarely clinical
Prognosis	3% to 10% mortality	10% to 20% mortality
Subsequent course	Insulin therapy required in virtually all cases	Insulin therapy not required in many cases

Abbreviations: DKA, diabetic ketoacidosis; HHNS, hyperglycemic hyperosmolar nonketotic syndrome.

Reprinted with permission from Peragallo-Dittko V, ed. *A Core Curriculum for Diabetes Education*, 2nd ed. Chicago: American Association of Diabetes Educators; 1993:326.

- Decreased mentation (mild confusion, lethargy) and lack of normal responsiveness are common and correlate best with serum osmolality. These are the usual reasons that patients with HHNS seek medical attention.
- Focal neurologic signs may be present and may mimic a cerebrovascular event (hemisensory deficits, hemiparesis, aphasia, seizures); these signs decline as biochemical status returns to normal.

A diagnosis of HHNS usually is made easily if one has a high index of suspicion. Patients may be admitted to the neurology or neurosurgical service because only neurologic conditions are considered initially. Routine urine and blood tests can help clarify the diagnosis of HHNS. Health care professionals need to be alert for signs of HHNS in patients at chronic-care facilities because this diagnosis tends to be overlooked in such settings.

Laboratory Evaluation

Typical laboratory values in HHNS are shown in Table 11.3.

Treatment

Lifesaving measures may be needed immediately. The primary treatment goal is rehydration to restore circulating plasma volume and correct electrolyte deficits. In addition, the precipitating event should be identified and corrected, and other goals similar to those described for treatment of DKA should be instituted, including providing adequate insulin to restore and maintain normal glucose metabolism. Glucose concentration is the major biochemical end point because patients with HHNS do not have ketosis or acidosis.

- Cardiovascular status should be monitored closely and frequently during fluid replacement to avoid precipitating congestive heart failure, given the fact that most patients with HHNS are older and have preexisting heart disease.
- Insulin is administered in the same manner as for patients with DKA. At glucose concentrations of 250 mg/dL, the rate of insulin infusion should be decreased to 2 to 3 U/h and dextrose should be added to the IV fluid because oral intake will not be possible for many hours to a few days.
- Dextrose (50 g) should be given intravenously every 8 hours and insulin dose adjusted accordingly (decreased 1 to 3 U/h) based on plasma glucose measurements every 4 hours.
- Potassium replacement follows the same guidelines as for DKA, with consideration of the special conditions of patients with HHNS (underlying renal disease is associated with lower urinary potassium losses, preexisting heart disease is associated with greater susceptibility to the effects of potassium).
- Bicarbonate therapy is contraindicated in absence of acidosis.
- Phosphate replacement follows the same guidelines as for DKA, with consideration of the effect of phosphate on underlying renal disease.

11

■ Hypoglycemia

This metabolic problem occurs in both type 1 and less commonly in type 2 diabetes when there is an imbalance between food intake and the appropriate dosage and timing of drug therapy (oral agents, insulin). Other factors that contribute to hypoglycemia are:

- Exercise
- Alcohol intake
- Other drugs
- Decreased liver or kidney function.

Signs of Hypoglycemia

The incidence of hypoglycemia in patients with type 2 diabetes is several orders of magnitude lower than in type 1 diabetes. Nonetheless, patients taking insulin, sulfonylureas, and/or glinides are prone to hypoglycemia.

Hypoglycemia should be suspected in patients who demonstrate the following clinical signs; a diagnosis of hypoglycemia is confirmed in a symptomatic patient if a plasma glucose level <60 mg/dL (<3.3 mM) is found:

- Mild hypoglycemia is associated with adrenergic or cholinergic symptoms such as:
  - Pallor
  - Diaphoresis
  - Tachycardia
  - Palpitations
  - Hunger
  - Paresthesias
  - Shakiness
- Moderate hypoglycemia (<40 mg/dL) is associated with neuroglycopenic symptoms of altered mental and/or neurologic functioning such as:
  - Inability to concentrate
  - Confusion
  - Slurred speech
  - Irrational or uncontrolled behavior
  - Slowed reaction time
  - Blurred vision
  - Somnolence
  - Extreme fatigue
- Severe hypoglycemia (<20 mg/dL) is associated with extreme impairment of neurologic function to the extent that the assistance of another person is needed to obtain treatment; symptoms include:
  - Completely automatic/disoriented behavior
  - Loss of consciousness

– Inability to arouse from sleep
– Seizures
- Nocturnal hypoglycemia is associated with over 50% of cases of severe hypoglycemia; early symptoms do not awaken patients and the predinner intermediate-acting insulins may cause hyperinsulinemia and hypoglycemia in the early morning hours.

It is important to understand that hypoglycemia does not necessarily progress in a linear fashion from mild to severe. For example, some patients might develop neuroglycopenic symptoms before adrenergic or cholinergic symptoms, and other patients may overlook or ignore adrenergic or cholinergic symptoms and progress to neuroglycopenia.

Treatment
The goal of treatment is to normalize the plasma glucose level as quickly as possible.
- Mild hypoglycemia is treated most effectively by having the patient ingest approximately 15 g of readily available carbohydrate by mouth. Sources of carbohydrate (15 g) include:
  – Three glucose tablets (5 g each)
  – $^1/_2$ cup fruit juice
  – 2 tablespoons raisins
  – Five Lifesavers® candy
  – $^1/_2$ to $^3/_4$ cup regular soda (not diet)
  – 1 cup milk
  If symptoms continue, treatment may need to be repeated in 15 minutes. Most patients can resume normal activity following treatment.
- For moderate hypoglycemia, larger amounts of carbohydrate (15 to 30 g) that are rapidly absorbed may be needed. Patients usually are instructed to consume additional food after the initial treatment and wait approximately 30

11

205

minutes until resuming activity. Measuring blood glucose levels during treatment and the recovery periods can help determine the effectiveness of treatment. Some patients, however, may continue to have neuroglycopenic symptoms for an hour or longer after blood glucose levels have increased to above 100 mg/dL.

- Severe hypoglycemia requires rapid treatment. IV glucose (50 cc 50% dextrose or glucose followed by 10% dextrose drip) is the most effective route; however, glucagon (1 mg for adults) can be administered IM at home with positive results. Individuals who are unable to swallow should be given glucose gel, honey, syrup, or jelly on the inside of the cheek. After the initial response, a rapid-acting, carbohydrate-containing liquid should be given until nausea subsides; then a small snack or meal can be consumed. Blood glucose levels should be monitored frequently for several hours to assure that the levels remain normal and to avoid overtreatment. The individual's health care team should be informed of any severe hypoglycemic episodes.

Prevention of Hypoglycemia

Patients can take certain measures to avoid hypoglycemia:

- Know the signs and symptoms of hypoglycemia.
- Try to eat meals on a regular schedule.
- Carry a source of carbohydrate (at least 10 to 15 g).
- Perform self-monitoring blood glucose (SMBG) regularly for early detection of low blood glucose levels; initiate treatment at the first signs of hypoglycemia.
- Take regular insulin at least 30 minutes before eating. (Patients who take their regular insulin

immediately before or after the meal will be prone to delayed hypoglycemia.) A fast-acting insulin analog should be taken 5 minutes before consumption of the meal.

- Schedule exercise appropriately; adjust meal times, calorie intake, or insulin dosing to accommodate physical activity; use SMBG (before, during, after strenuous activity) to determine the effect of exercise on blood glucose levels and to detect low blood glucose levels.
- Check blood glucose level before going to sleep to avoid nocturnal hypoglycemia; perform nocturnal (3:00 AM) monitoring:
  - If hypoglycemia has occurred during the night
  - When evening insulin has been adjusted
  - When strenuous activity has occurred the previous day
  - During times of irregular eating schedules or erratic glucose control
- Several nutrition bars that are low in fat have been developed to help prevent hypoglycemia (Extend Bar).

Infection

Infection is the primary cause of metabolic abnormalities leading to diabetic coma in patients with diabetes. Because of the potentially severe consequences of untreated infections, prompt diagnosis and treatment is essential. Infections are often occult in diabetic patients and require a high index of suspicion. Common infections in patients with diabetes are shown in Table 11.4.

TABLE 11.4 — INFECTIONS COMMON OR SPECIAL TO PATIENTS WITH DIABETES MELLITUS	
Type of Infection	**Comments**
Cutaneous Furunculosis Carbuncles	For reasons not clear, patients with diabetes mellitus may be prone to recurrent furunculosis and carbuncles. Unless vascular insufficiency is present, warm compresses may be used for treatment. Antibiotics are sometimes needed with and without drainage.
Vulvovaginitis (less frequently, scrotal infections)	*Candida* skin infection commonly occurs in warm, moist areas, particularly in the region of the genitalia (also on the inner thighs and under the breasts). This is particularly common in people with type 2 diabetes who are overweight, have poor metabolic control, or who have been taking antibiotics. These infections can cause extreme discomfort to the patient and result in breakdown of skin, which may allow entry of more virulent organisms. Good glycemic control and local supportive antifungal treatment usually will resolve the problem. Occasionally, oral antifungal therapy is needed.

Cellulitis, alone or in combination with lower extremity vascular ulcers	To prevent the spread of infection to bone and the necessity of amputation, treatment of infected ulcers and surrounding cellulitis must be aggressive. Antibiotics effective against bacteria recovered from the site (both aerobes and anaerobes should be expected) should be used, as well as surgical debridement and drainage.
Urinary tract	Asymptomatic bacteriuria occurs in up to 20% of patients with diabetes mellitus; some suggest that it be treated. Certainly, a patient with neurogenic bladder is susceptible to urinary tract infection and sepsis. Treatment is mandatory in patients with pyelonephritis. Patients with serious urinary tract infections should be hospitalized, the offending pathogens identified, and appropriate susceptibility tests performed.
Ear	Malignant external otitis is relatively rare, but when it occurs, it is most often seen in elderly diabetic patients with chronically draining ear and sudden onset of severe pain. *Pseudomonas aeruginosa* is the usual pathogenic organism. This condition is fatal in ~50% of cases. Immediate treatment should include appropriate antibiotic therapy and surgical debridement when indicated.

Reprinted with permission from American Diabetes Association. *Medical Management of Type 2 Diabetes*, 5th ed. Alexandria, Va: American Diabetes Association; 1999.

11

Quality of Life

Patients with blood glucose values consistently greater than 200 mg/dL will have a reduced quality of life. Poorly controlled blood glucose values will lead to excessive thirst and urination, causing nocturia and poor sleep. Poor sleep will lead to daytime tiredness and poor work performance in adults. Patients will have frequent urinary tract infections, tooth and gum disease and blurry vision. It has also been shown that the elderly experience cognitive impairment and a higher incidence of falls.

SUGGESTED READING

Peragallo-Dittko V, ed. *A Core Curriculum for Diabetes Education*, 2nd ed. Chicago, Ill: American Association of Diabetes Educators; 1993.

Porte D, Sherwin RS. *Ellenburg & Rifkin's Diabetes Mellitus*. 5th ed. Stamford, Conn: Appleton & Lange; 1997.

12 Long-Term Complications

The long-term complications that may develop in patients with type 2 diabetes include:
- Macrovascular disease
- Microvascular disease:
  – Diabetic retinopathy
  – Diabetic nephropathy
  – Diabetic neuropathy:
    - Symmetric distal neuropathy
    - Mononeuropathy
    - Diabetic amyotrophy
    - Gastroparesis
    - Diabetic diarrhea
    - Neurogenic bladder
    - Impaired cardiovascular reflexes (sudden death)
    - Sexual dysfunction
- Diabetic foot disorders.

The long-term, chronic complications of diabetes have the greatest impact on the health of individuals with diabetes as well as on the healthcare system. Diabetes and its associated vascular complications are the fourth leading cause of death in the United States. Consequently, early detection and aggressive treatment of these complications are essential to reduce associated morbidity and mortality. Striving for tight metabolic control also has been proven to help delay the onset and prevent the development of microvascular complications (diabetic retinopathy, nephropathy, and neuropathy).

The Diabetes Control and Complications Trial (DCCT), a multicenter, randomized clinical trial, investigated the effects of intensive therapy versus traditional therapy on the development and progression of microvascular complications of type 1 diabetes mellitus. The aim of intensive therapy was to achieve and maintain near-normal blood glucose values following a regimen of three or more daily insulin injections or treatment with an insulin pump. In contrast, only one or two insulin injections were used in conventional therapy. Patients were followed for a mean of 6.5 years and assessed regularly for the presence or progression of retinopathy, nephropathy, and neuropathy.

Intensive therapy proved to be highly effective in delaying the onset and slowing the progression of the long-term complications being evaluated in patients with type 1 diabetes. Furthermore, similar benefits were observed in the United Kingdom Prospective Diabetes Study (UKPDS) in type 2 diabetes. In response to the DCCT and UKPDS findings, the American Diabetes Association recommended striving for the best possible glycemic control in patients with type 1 and type 2 diabetes, with the following goals:

- Fasting and preprandial blood glucose level of 80 mg/dL to 120 mg/dL
- Postprandial glucose level of less than 160 mg/dL
- Glycosylated hemoglobin of <7% (normal reference range = 4% to 6%) or three standard deviations from the mean of the normal range.

Attempts to normalize glycemia and glycosylated hemoglobin should be balanced, however, with minimizing weight gain and hypoglycemia, and maintaining an acceptable quality of life.

Macrovascular Disease

The incidence of the three major macrovascular diseases (coronary artery, cerebrovascular, and peripheral vascular) is greater in individuals with diabetes than in nondiabetic individuals, accounting for up to 80% of mortality in adults with diabetes. Atherosclerosis develops at an earlier age, accelerates more rapidly, and is more extensive in patients with diabetes than in nondiabetics matched by age, weight, and sex.

Type 2 diabetes is a risk factor for macrovascular disease as are conditions that commonly coexist in patients with diabetes (hypertension, dyslipidemia, and central obesity). Smoking and lack of exercise contribute to an increased risk in both type 2 diabetes and the nondiabetic population. In addition, renal insufficiency can increase the risk of and accelerate macrovascular disease in diabetic individuals with microalbuminuria or gross proteinuria.

Weight control and exercise are safe and effective methods for modifying macrovascular risk and should form the basis to which all other treatments are added. The following treatments for hypertension and dyslipidemia should be applied where appropriate.

■ Hypertension

Hypertension should be treated vigorously in all patients with diabetes to limit and/or prevent the development and progression of atherosclerosis, nephropathy, and retinopathy. Lowering elevated blood pressure is the most important and immediate consideration, with a therapeutic goal of <130/85 mm Hg if there is no evidence of protein in the urine. The goal for patients with isolated systolic hypertension (180 mm Hg) is 160 mm Hg; further reductions to 140 mm Hg are suggested if the treatment is well tolerated. The goal for patients with renal insufficiency should be <120/80 mm Hg with a mean blood pressure <93 mm Hg.

Treatment should be initiated with a no-added salt diet and weight loss (for obese patients) combined with appropriate aerobic exercise. Because patients with diabetes can be uniquely impacted by certain side effects of antihypertensives, physicians must be familiar with the potential complications of the classes of antihypertensive drugs (Table 12.1).

In general, reductions in systolic or diastolic blood pressure of 5% to 10% occur with most antihypertensives. The potential benefits of the commonly prescribed antihypertensives are shown in Table 12.2. Treatment guidelines include:

- One or more antihypertensive medications may be necessary to achieve satisfactory blood pressure control.
- Adding a second drug to small or moderate doses of the first drug often results in better control with fewer side effects than using full doses of the first agent.

Angiotensin-Converting Enzyme Inhibitors

Angiotensin-converting enzyme (ACE) inhibitors and now the angiotensin-receptor blockers (ARBs) commonly are the first choices for therapy because they are effective and have a low incidence of side effects. They are useful in diabetic patients with and without nephropathy. In the UKPDS, the ACE inhibitor captopril was equally efficacious as the β-blocker atenolol in reducing microvascular and cardiovascular complications of type 2 diabetes. They have no negative impact on carbohydrate or lipid metabolism, can slow the rate of progression of proteinuria in diabetic nephropathy, reduce the decline in renal function, and prevent progression of retinopathy. Caution should be used in patients with peripheral occlusive disease because renal artery stenosis may be present, which could lead to renal decline with ACE inhibitors.

ACE inhibitors have now been shown to be cardioprotective in addition to their beneficial effects on the diabetic kidney. The Health Outcomes Prevention Evaluation (HOPE) trial studied over 3500 subjects with diabetes who had documentation of previ-

TABLE 12.1 — POTENTIAL COMPLICATIONS OF COMMON ANTIHYPERTENSIVE AGENTS IN THE PATIENT WITH DIABETES

Drug	Potential Complications
Angiotensin-converting enzyme inhibitors	Proteinuria (can occur in patients with severe bilateral renal artery stenosis), reduced renal function, hyperkalemia, cough, leukopenia/agranulocytosis (rare)
Angiotensin receptor blockers	Have the same renal-protective effects as ACE inhibitors; they do not cause cough but can cause hyperkalemia
β-*Adrenergic blockers*	
Nonselective β$_1$- and β$_2$-blockers	Cardiac failure, impaired insulin release with hyperglycemia, hypoglycemia unawareness, delayed recovery from hyperglycemia, impotence
Cardioselective (cardioselectivity may be lost with high doses) β$_1$-blockers	Blunted symptoms of hypoglycemia, hypertension associated with hypoglycemia, hyperlipidemia, impotence
α-Blockers	Orthostatic hypotension
Calcium channel blockers	Pedal edema, constipation, heart block, negative inotropic effect (depending on agent selected)
Thiazide and loop diuretics	Hypokalemia, hyperglycemia, dyslipidemia, impotence

	TABLE 12.2 — POTENTIAL BENEFITS OF COMMON ANTIHYPERTENSIVE AGENTS		
Class	**Effects on Coronary Events Rates**	**Effects on Progression of Renal Disease**	**Effects on Stroke**
ACE inhibitors	Beneficial	Beneficial	Beneficial
ARBs	Unknown	Beneficial	Unknown
β-Blockers	Beneficial	Beneficial	Beneficial
α-Blockers	Controversial	Unknown	Unknown
CCBs	Controversial	Controversial	Beneficial
NDCCBs	Unknown	Beneficial	Unknown
Thiazide diuretics	Beneficial	Unknown	Beneficial
Loop diuretics	Unknown	Unknown	Unknown

Abbreviations: ACE, angiotensin-converting enzyme; ARB, angiotensin II receptor blocker; CCB, calcium channel blocker; NDCCB, nondihydropyridine calcium channel blocker.

Adapted from: ADA Clinical Practice Recommendations. *Diabetes Care.* 2002;25:137.

ous cardiovascular events and were over 55 years of age. Subjects were randomized to either ramipril (10 mg/day) or placebo and vitamin E or placebo. Within 4.5 years, the ramipril-treated group experienced a 22% reduction in myocardial infarction, a 33% reduction in stroke, a 37% reduction in any cardiovascular event, and a 24% reduction in the development of overt nephropathy when compared with the placebo group. These benefits occurred despite minor reductions in blood pressure, raising the possibility that ACE inhibitors have benefits for diabetic patients independent of blood pressure lowering. In summary, the HOPE study is a landmark study confirming the results of multiple smaller and less powered studies demonstrating the cardiac and renal protective effects of ACE inhibitors in subjects with diabetes. Based on the results of these studies, ACE inhibitors should be considered as first-line therapy in diabetics with mild to moderate hypertension and/or micro- or macroalbuminuria.

Serum potassium should be monitored during therapy with ACE inhibitors in patients with suspected hyporeninemic hypoaldosteronism (type IV renal tubular acidosis) to prevent severe hyperkalemia.

Angiotensin II Receptor Blockers

Like the ACE inhibitors, ARBs have been shown to slow the progression of albuminuria and be protective in diabetic nephropathy. There is some evidence from the Candesartan and Lisinopril Microalbuminuria (CALM) study that combining an ACE inhibitor and ARB reduces blood pressure and urinary albumin levels more than either agent alone.

β-*Blockers*

β-Blockers are being used more frequently as antihypertensive agents following the beneficial effects reported with atenolol in the UKPDS. Besides equal efficacy to the ACE inhibitor captopril, atenolol-treated patients did not have an increased incidence of hypoglycemic episodes. However, it is probably prudent to avoid β-blockers in patients with a history of severe hypoglycemia or hypoglycemic unawareness. The potential to blunt counter-regulatory responses or prolong hypoglycemia needs to be weighed against the clearcut benefits of β-blockers to reduce mortality in diabetic patients with recent myocardial infarction. Selective β-blockers may be more beneficial than the nonselective β-blockers, and have a lower incidence of side effects.

α-*Blockers*

α-Adrenergic blockers have been associated with improved insulin sensitivity and modest decreases in LDL cholesterol, but no long-term randomized studies have been conducted examining renal or cardiovascular outcomes. Orthostatic hypotension can occur, so caution should be used in patients with diabetic autonomic neuropathy.

Calcium Channel Blockers

There are three subclasses of calcium channel blockers: the dihydropyridine group (DCCBs) and the benzothiazepines and phenylalkylamines (NDCCBs). The DCCBs are a heterogenous class of compounds with significant pharmacologic differences and a primary vasodilatory effect. Due to conflicting evidence, it is unclear whether the DCCBs reduce cardiovascular events or progression of nephropathy. They may protect against stroke, but appear to be less effective than ACE inhibitors in reducing cardiovascular events. An increase in cardiovascular mortality has been reported with the short-acting DCCB nifedipine. Short-acting DCCBs are not approved and should not be used to treat hypertension in diabetic patients.

Use of the NDCCBs have been associated with decreased proteinuria in short-term studies of patients with overt diabetic nephropathy.

Diuretics

Low-dose thiazide diuretic use has been associated with reduced risk of congestive heart failure and stroke in large randomized trials. Treatment of systolic hypertension in older diabetic subjects with low-dose thiazides significantly reduced cardiovascular events. Their effects on progression of renal impairment have not been studied in large randomized clinical trials. Low-dose thiazides probably do not impair insulin sensitivity or worsen the lipid profile as high doses have been reported to do. Low-dose thiazide diuretics may be particularly useful in combination with other antihypertensive agents. The loop diuretics have been used in combination therapy, particularly in diabetic patients with decreased renal function.

■ Dyslipidemia

Lipid abnormalities that accelerate atherosclerosis and increase the risk of cardiovascular disease are significantly more common in patients with type 2 diabetes than in nondiabetic individuals. In addition, central obesity associated with type 2 diabetes is also a risk factor for cardiovascular disease. These combined factors have resulted in cardiovascular disease becoming a major cause of morbidity and mortality in type 2 diabetes.

The characteristic lipid abnormalities in type 2 diabetes are:

- Hypertriglyceridemia usually due to elevated triglyceride-rich, very low-density lipoprotein (VLDL) levels and sometimes increased chylomicrons as well

12

- Decreased high-density lipoprotein (HDL) levels
- Phenotype B pattern (excessive amounts of small, dense low-density lipoprotein [LDL] and intermediate-density lipoprotein [IDL] particles), which contribute to an increased cardiovascular risk.

Given this higher risk of premature cardiovascular disease in type 2 diabetes, all patients should be screened for lipid abnormalities at the initial evaluation using a fasting lipid profile to determine serum triglyceride, total cholesterol, HDL cholesterol, and LDL cholesterol levels. Shown in Table 12.3 are acceptable, borderline, and high-risk lipid levels for adults. LDL cholesterol is calculated from the formula:

$$LDL = \text{total cholesterol} - HDL - (\text{triglycerides} \div 5)$$

This calculation is not accurate if the triglycerides are greater than 400 mg/dL and LDL should be measured directly by ultracentrifugation. The recommendations for the treatment decisions based on elevated LDL are shown in Table 12.4. Pharmacologic therapy should be initiated after nutrition and behavioral interventions. However, when clinical cardiovascular disease is present or LDL is very high ($\geq$200 mg/dL), pharmacologic therapy should be initiated at the same time.

Because lipid abnormalities often reflect poor glycemic control, the first treatment approach to dyslipidemia in type 2 diabetes should be optimizing diabetes control with diet, exercise, and pharmacologic therapy as needed. As glycemic control improves, lipid levels also usually improve, particularly when insulin resistance is the underlying metabolic abnormality responsible for the lipid disorder.

Limiting calories and saturated fat intake have proved to be highly effective in improving, but not

220

TABLE 12.3 — LIPID LEVELS FOR ADULTS

Risk for Adult Diabetic Patients	Cholesterol (mg/dL)	HDL Cholesterol* (mg/dL)	LDL Cholesterol (mg/dL)	Triglycerides (mg/dL)
Low	<200	>45	<100	<200
Borderline	200–239	35–45	100–129	200–399
High	≥240	<35	≥130	≥400

* For women, the HDL cholesterol values should be increased by 10 mg/dL.

American Diabetes Association. Clinical practice recommendations 2002. Management of dyslipidemia in adults with diabetes. *Diabetes Care*. 2002;25(suppl 1):S74-S77.

12

TABLE 12.4 — TREATMENT DECISIONS BASED ON LDL CHOLESTEROL LEVEL IN ADULTS WITH DIABETES

Risk Factors	Medical Nutrition Therapy		Drug Therapy	
	Initiation Level (mg/dL)	LDL Goal (mg/dL)	Initiation Level (mg/dL)	LDL Goal (mg/dL)
With CHD, PVD, or CVD	≥100	<100	≥100	<100
Without CHD, PVD, or CVD	≥100	<100	≥130*	<100

Abbreviations: CHD, coronary heart disease; CVD, cardiovascular disease; HDL, high-density lipoprotein; LDL, low-density lipoprotein; PVD, peripheral vascular disease.

* For patients with LDL between 100 and 129 mg/dL, a variety of treatment strategies are available, including more aggressive nutrition therapy and pharmacological treatment with a statin; in addition, if the HDL is <40 mg/dL, a fibric acid such as fenofibrate may be used in these patients. Nutrition therapy should be attempted before starting pharmacological therapy.

Diabetes Care. 2002;25(suppl 1):S75.

usually normalizing, the dyslipidemia of type 2 diabetes. Increased intake of soluble fiber, particularly from oat and bean products, has been shown to reduce LDL cholesterol levels. The National Cholesterol Education Program (NCEP) has designed a stepped approach for restricting dietary fat and cholesterol that can be modified to incorporate specific requirements for diabetic nutrition. The following guidelines should be implemented with the assistance of a registered dietitian:

- Step 1 diet guidelines: limit saturated fat intake to 8% to 10% of daily calories, with 30% of calories from total fat; limit cholesterol to <300 mg cholesterol per day. If this approach is not adequate for meeting lipid goals, initiate Step 2.
- Step 2 diet guidelines: limit saturated fat intake to <7% of daily calories; limit cholesterol intake to <200 mg/day.
- If triglycerides are >1000 mg/dL, all dietary fats should be reduced to lower circulating chylomicrons.

Recommendations for effective diet therapy for the treatment of lipid disorders in diabetes are shown in Table 12.5.

Lipid-lowering pharmacologic agents are usually necessary when the lipid profile does not normalize in response to diet, exercise, and efforts to improve glycemic control. The American Diabetes Association follows an order of priority for the treatment of diabetic dyslipidemia (Table 12.6). LDL cholesterol is considered the first priority, followed by HDL cholesterol raising, triglyceride lowering, and treatment of combined hyperlipidemia. Commonly used pharmacologic agents for the treatment of dyslipidemia are listed in Table 12.7:

- When elevated LDL cholesterol is the primary lipoprotein abnormality: HMG-CoA reductase

TABLE 12.5 — DIET RECOMMENDATIONS FOR THE TREATMENT OF LIPID DISORDERS IN DIABETES

- Calorie restriction and increased physical activity for weight loss as indicated
- Saturated and trans-unsaturated fat intake <10% and preferably <7% of total energy intake
- Total dietary cholesterol intake <200 mg/day
- Emphasis on complex carbohydrates (at least five portions per day of fruits/vegetables); soluble fibers (legumes, oats, certain fruits/vegetables) have additional benefits on total cholesterol, LDL cholesterol level, and glycemic control
- Replacing saturated fat with carbohydrate or monounsaturated fats (eg, canola oil, olive oil)

inhibitors (atorvastatin, fluvastatin, lovastatin, pravastatin, simvastatin) are indicated. These agents reduce cholesterol synthesis and are useful as monotherapy for the familial forms of hypercholesterolemia, or in combination with bile acid sequestrants. Most HMG-CoA reductase inhibitors are indicated for the reduction of both LDL cholesterol and triglyceride levels. When serum triglycerides are consistently elevated above 200 mg/dL, with or without low HDL levels, medication is warranted in addition to a low-fat diet.

- Bile acid sequestrants (Colestid, Questran) have several disadvantages in patients with diabetes. Bile binders must be taken 1 hour before or 4 hours after other oral medications so there is no interference with absorption. Bile binders also cause fairly significant constipation, and this is especially bothersome in the diabetic population because it exacerbates the constipation of diabetic gastroparesis. In addition, bile

TABLE 12.6 — ORDER OF PRIORITIES FOR TREATMENT OF DIABETIC DYSLIPIDEMIA IN ADULTS*

- LDL cholesterol lowering*:
  - First choice: HMG CoA reductase inhibitor (statin)
  - Second choice: bile acid binding resin (resin) or fenofibrate
- HDL cholesterol raising:
  - Behavioral interventions such as weight loss, increased physical activity, and smoking cessation may be useful
  - Difficult except with nicotinic acid, which should be used with caution, or fibrates
- Triglyceride lowering:
  - Glycemic control first priority
  - Fibric acid derivative (gemfibrozil, fenofibrate)
  - Statins are moderately effective at high dose in hyper-triglyceridemic subjects who also have high LDL cholesterol
- Combined hyperlipidemia:
  - First choice: improved glycemic control plus high-dose statin
  - Second choice: improved glycemic control plus statin[†] plus fibric acid derivative[†] (gemfibrozil, fenofibrate)
  - Third choice: Improved glycemic control plus resin plus fibric acid derivative (gemfibrozil, fenofibrate); or improved glycemic control plus statin[†] plus nicotinic acid[†] (glycemic control must be monitored carefully)

Abbreviations: HDL, high-density lipoprotein; HMG CoA, 3-hydroxy-3-methylglutaryl coenzyme A; LDL, low-density lipoprotein.

* Decision for treatment of high LDL before elevated triglyceride is based on clinical trial data indicating safety as well as efficacy of the available agents.
† The combination of statins with nicotinic acid and especially with gemfibrozil or fenofibrate may carry an increased risk of myositis.

Diabetes Care. 2002;25(suppl 1):S76.

12

TABLE 12.7 — PHARMACOLOGIC AGENTS FOR TREATMENT OF DYSLIPIDEMIA IN ADULTS

	Agent	Effect on Lipoprotein			Clinical Trials in Diabetic Subjects
		LDL	HDL	Triglyceride	
First-Line	LDL lowering				
	HMG-CoA reductase inhibitor	↓↓	↔↑	↔↓	4S (simvastatin); CARE (pravastatin)
	Triglyceride lowering				
	Fibric acid derivative	↓↔↑	↑	↓↓	Helsinki (gemfibrozil)
Second-Line	LDL lowering				
	Bile acid binding resins	↓	↔	↑	None
	LDL and triglyceride lowering				
	Nicotinic acid*	↓	↑↑	↓↓	None

Abbreviations: 4S, Scandinavian Simvastatin Survival Study; CARE, Cholesterol and Recurrent Events; HDL, high-density lipoprotein; HMG-CoA, 3-hydroxy-3-methylglutaryl coenzyme A; LDL, low-density lipoprotein.

* In diabetic patients, nicotinic acid should be restricted to ≤2 g/d; short-acting nicotinic acid is preferred.

Diabetes Care. 2002;25(suppl 1):S77.

binders also can worsen hypertriglyceridemia in patients with diabetes.

- Nicotinic acid is highly effective at improving all lipoprotein parameters, although it significantly worsens glucose intolerance and is contraindicated in most patients with type 2 diabetes. Niaspan is a new slow-release niacin preparation that may be tolerated in a subset of severe dyslipidemic individuals with diabetes.

- Despite earlier warnings that HMG-CoA reductase inhibitors should not be used with gemfibrozil (Lopid) or fenofibrate (Tricor) in patients with mixed disorders, they offer a safe and effective approach to diabetic patients with elevated triglycerides and LDL cholesterol values. When adding one medication to the other, creatinine phosphokinase (CPK) should be measured and liver function tests should be performed in 3 weeks and again in 6 weeks, along with a lipoprotein profile. Once a stable dose is maintained and the CPK and liver function tests are below three times the upper limit of normal, then monitoring these values frequently becomes unnecessary. Caution should be used if the patient is on other medications that could cause hepatitis or myositis. Lastly, this combination should only be used in compliant patients who will not get lost to medical follow-up.

- When hypertriglyceridemia is the primary lipid abnormality (triglyceride levels consistently >200 mg/dL with or without low HDL levels), a fibric acid derivative is the drug of choice; gemfibrozil reduces triglyceride levels usually with small decreases in LDL cholesterol and small increases in HDL cholesterol. Fenofibrate is a fenofibric acid derivative that may lower LDL cholesterol in addition to reducing triglyceride values and increasing

12

HDL levels. These agents are particularly effective at decreasing hepatic VLDL production and enhancing the clearance of VLDL triglycerides by stimulating lipoprotein lipase (LPL) and are well tolerated.

- Low HDL levels are extremely difficult to treat. Nicotinic acid can be of benefit but often leads to deterioration in glucose control. Fibrates also improve HDL modestly. Perhaps the best medications to increase HDL in type 2 diabetic subjects are the glitazones which can increase HDL up to 20%.

- An effective therapeutic option for combined dyslipidemia is the use of an HMG-CoA reductase inhibitor which is indicated for the treatment of elevated LDL cholesterol and triglyceride levels. LDL cholesterol can be reduced up to 60% and triglycerides up to 40% with HMG-CoA reductase inhibitors.

Microvascular Complications

Retinopathy, nephropathy, and neuropathy are the major microvascular complications of type 2 diabetes. Prevention, early detection, and aggressive treatment are essential to reduce associated morbidity and mortality. Good metabolic control has been clearly shown to prevent the development and delay the progression of these complications in both types of diabetes.

■ Diabetic Retinopathy

The development and progression of retinopathy depends on the duration of diabetes and the duration and severity of hyperglycemia. Because diabetic retinopathy does not cause symptoms until it has reached an advanced stage, early and frequent evaluation for vision problems is critical for patients with diabetes. The following findings also support the importance of early detection:

- Diabetes is the leading cause of all new cases of blindness (13%).
- Loss of vision associated with diabetic retinopathy and macular edema can be reduced by at least 50% with laser photocoagulation if identified in a timely manner.

Patients must be completely informed about the possible relationship between hyperglycemia and retinopathy, stressing the importance of promptly reporting any visual symptoms. They should be aware that hypertension can worsen retinopathy and therefore be encouraged to take any antihypertensive medications that have been prescribed. Most importantly, patients should understand the potential visual complications associated with diabetic retinopathy and how to prevent or reduce the severity of these problems.

The three categories of diabetic retinopathy that are part of a continuum are:

- Nonproliferative or background
- Preproliferative
- Proliferative.

Nonproliferative

Background changes are the earliest stage of retinopathy and are characterized by microaneurysms and intraretinal "dot and blot" hemorrhages (Figure 12.1). If serous fluid leaks into the area of the maculae (where central vision originates), macular edema can occur and cause disruption in light transmission and visual acuity. Macular edema cannot be observed directly but is suggested by the presence of hard exudates close to the maculae. Any of these findings should prompt immediate referral to an ophthalmologist.

FIGURE 12.1 — BACKGROUND DIABETIC RETINOPATHY

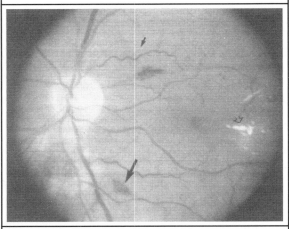

Note microaneurysm (short dark arrow), hard exudate (open arrow), and hemorrhage (long dark arrow).

Courtesy of Albert Sheffer, MD.

Preproliferative

Advanced background retinopathy with certain lesions is considered the preproliferative stage and indicates an increased risk of progression to proliferative retinopathy. This stage is characterized by "beading" of the retinal veins; soft exudates (also called "cotton-wool" spots that are ischemic infarcts of the inner retinal layers) (Figure 12.2); and irregular, dilated, and tortuous retinal capillaries or occasionally newly formed intraretinal vessels. Any of these signs suggests the need for further evaluation by an ophthalmologist.

Proliferative

Proliferative retinopathy is the final stage of this degenerative condition and imparts the most serious

FIGURE 12.2 — PREPROLIFERATIVE RETINOPATHY

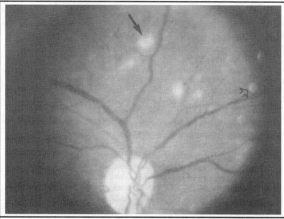

The soft or cotton wool exudate (dark arrow) has indistinct margins in contrast to the hard exudate in Figure 12.1, which has sharp margins and is brighter. The round structures with distinct margins (open arrow) are artifacts.

Courtesy of Albert Sheffer, MD.

threat to vision. Neovascularization typically covers more than one third of the optic disk and may extend into the posterior vitreous. These fragile new vessels, which are prone to bleeding, probably develop in response to ischemia. Bleeding that occurs in the vitreous or preretinal space can cause visual symptoms such as "floaters" or "cobwebs," or retinal detachment that results from contraction of fibrous tissue. Sudden and painless vision loss usually is related to a major retinal hemorrhage.

Evaluation and Referral

Because visual acuity frequently changes in response to fluctuations in glycemic control (particularly extreme variations, eg, low-to-high and high-to-low), the reason for any vision changes should be thoroughly investigated. All patients with diabetes should have annual eye examinations with complete visual history, visual acuity examinations, and careful ophthalmoscopic examinations with a dilated pupil. Indications for referral to an ophthalmologist are shown in Table 12.8. Patients with type 1 diabetes should begin having annual eye examinations after 5 years of diabetes. Patients with type 2 diabetes should have annual eye examinations starting at the time of diagnosis because of the probability that glucose intolerance was present for up to 4 to 7 years before the diagnosis of diabetes.

Treatment

Treatment of nonproliferative and preproliferative retinopathy typically involves blood glucose control and blood pressure control. The only standard treatment for background retinopathy, in addition to optimizing metabolic control and blood pressure, is photocoagulation treatment. Results of the Early Treatment Diabetic Retinopathy Study (ETDRS) revealed the effectiveness of argon laser photocoagulation applied focally (eg, spot-welding the leaking microaneurysms) in treating macular edema and stabilizing vision. Photocoagulation can slow the progression of vision loss in cases of macular edema and reduce visual loss by more than 50% when used as a preventive measure to limit neovascularization and vitreous hemorrhages. Pan-retinal laser treatment has been proven effective and is the treatment of choice for patients with proliferative retinopathy and high-risk characteristics. A scatter pattern of 1200 to 1600 burns are applied throughout the periphery of the retina, avoiding the macular area.

Vitrectomy may be required to treat retinal detachment and large vitreous hemorrhages. This pro-

TABLE 12.8 — REASONS TO REFER PATIENTS WITH TYPE 2 DIABETES MELLITUS TO AN EYE DOCTOR

Asymptomatic Patients
Annual examinations are imperative
- Hard exudates near macula
- Any preproliferative or proliferative characteristics
- Pregnancy (prior to conception and during first trimester)

Symptomatic Patients
Annual examinations
- Blurry vision persisting for >1 to 2 days when not associated with a change in blood glucose
- Sudden loss of vision in one or both eyes
- Black spots, cobwebs, or flashing lights in field of vision

High-Risk Patients
Annual examinations
- Neovascularization covering more than one third of optic disk
- Vitreous or preretinal hemorrhage with any neovascularization, particularly on optic disk
- Macular edema

American Diabetes Association. Clinical Practice Recommendations 2002. *Diabetes Care*. 2002;25(suppl 1):S90.

cedure generally is reserved for patients with poor vision in whom the benefits outweigh the risks.

■ Diabetic Nephropathy

Over 20% of adults who have had diabetes for 20 years or more have clinically apparent nephropathy. This disease is progressive, takes years to develop, and requires laboratory evaluation for early detection because it generally is asymptomatic in the early stages.

Structural and functional changes in the kidneys occur early in the course of poorly controlled diabetes but do not produce clinical symptoms. The first sign of nephropathy is microalbuminuria (30 to 300 mg albumin/24 hours), which may be apparent at the time of diagnosis in patients with type 2 diabetes. The presence of microalbuminuria is not only a predictable marker of early diabetic nephropathy, but is also very strongly associated with coronary artery disease in patients with type 2 diabetes. In addition, hyperfiltration, indicated by an elevated creatinine clearance, is also a finding in early diabetic nephropathy. The important clinical point is that in this early stage of nephropathy, aggressive management may reverse or completely stabilize any abnormalities. Overt nephropathy is defined as urinary protein excretion >0.5 g/24 hours and clinical proteinuria characterized by albumin excretion rates >300 mg (0.3 g)/24 hours, typically accompanied by hypertension. The following conditions play a role in the development and acceleration of renal insufficiency:

- Chronic uncontrolled hyperglycemia
- Hypertension (virtually all patients who develop nephropathy also have hypertension [SBP >135 mm Hg, DBP >85 mm Hg])
- Neurogenic bladder leading to hydronephrosis and infections
- Urinary tract infection and obstruction
- Nephrotoxic drugs (nonsteroidal anti-inflammatory drugs, chronic analgesic abuse, radiocontrast dyes [should be performed only when adequate hydration and diuresis can be assured and if no other diagnostic alternatives are available]).

Patients with diabetes often develop uremia at lower creatinine levels than patients with renal insufficiency resulting from other causes. Second, even with dialysis, the prognosis for patients with diabetes is worse than that for nondiabetic patients. Patients with diabetes tend to start dialysis earlier because they develop symptoms sooner than other patients with renal disease. Therefore, a renal transplant is the preferred method of treatment, if possible, at this stage.

Evaluation

A routine urinalysis should be done at the time of diagnosis and then yearly. If the urinalysis is positive for protein (>300 mg of albumin or macroalbuminuria), then a 24-hour quantitative measure along with a creatinine clearance is important to obtain. If the urinalysis is negative, then a test for microalbuminuria is indicated. The easiest method is the albumin to creatinine ratio in a random spot collection. The gold standard is a 24-hour collection and can be used to accurately follow the patient over time and assess the success of therapy. If a urinary tract infection is present it should be treated promptly before determining the significance of proteinuria. A positive result (>30 mg protein/24 hour) indicates the need for pharmacologic therapy with an ACE inhibitor or ARB.

Annual screening is important for patients who have negative results (particularly those without microalbuminuria and hypertension), given that certain factors can interfere transiently with this evaluation (eg, exercise, infections, fever, uncontrolled diabetes, hypertension). The mean albumin excretion of three timed urine collections can be used to establish a diagnosis of microalbuminuria if the values are equivocal.

It is important for physicians to inform patients with diabetes about the relationship between high blood pressure and renal disease, and the benefits of maintaining glycemic control. Patients should be encouraged to have their blood pressure checked regularly (in addition to obtaining their own blood pressure cuff to measure blood pressure at home), take antihypertensive medications that have been prescribed, decrease their protein intake to approximately 10% of daily calories, and monitor glucose levels frequently with self-monitoring of blood glucose (SMBG) and take any other measures to improve glycemia. The importance of reporting symptoms of urinary tract infection should be emphasized, along with following proper treatment for this infection and avoiding nephrotoxic drugs.

Treatment

Treatment is aimed at early detection and prevention, focusing specifically on improving glycemic control, aggressively treating hypertension (eg, with ACE inhibitor or ARB therapy and other agents as necessary), and restricting protein intake. If proteinuria is persistent or progressive, hypertension does not respond to treatment, or serum creatinine continues to be elevated, a nephrologist should be consulted. There is also evidence that treating an elevated LDL cholesterol level and taking antioxidants such as vitamin E and C, may be beneficial to the diabetic kidney.

Improving Glycemic Control

Considerable evidence supports the importance of optimizing glycemic control in delaying the development and slowing the progression of diabetic nephropathy. In the DCCT and UKPDS, intensive metabolic control was associated with a decrease in the development of microalbuminuria and clinical grade proteinuria in patients with type 1 and type 2 diabetes. The benefits of improved glycemia appear to be greatest before the onset of macroalbuminuria; once overt diabetic nephropathy has developed, improved glycemia has little beneficial effects on the progression of renal disease.

Research has revealed a glycemic threshhold for developing microalbuminuria, establishing a glycosylated hemoglobin level of <7% (normal is 4% to 6%) as the new glycemic goal whereas previously it was <8%. The risk of developing microalbuminuria is substantially reduced at this level.

Treating Hypertension

Controlling hypertension through aggressive therapeutic intervention can reduce proteinuria and considerably delay the progression of renal insufficiency. ACE inhibitors and ARBs offer effective antihypertensive effects in addition to significant delaying of the progression of diabetic nephropathy to end-stage renal disease. ACE inhibitors and ARBs decrease proteinuria by minimizing efferent glomerular vasoconstriction and reducing glomerular hyperfiltration. In cases where the glomerular filtration rate has already declined, ACE inhibitors also can partially reverse or prevent a further decrease. ACE inhibitors and ARBs should be considered as first-line therapy in all normotensive and hypertensive patients with diabetes who have microalbuminuria or macroalbuminuria. ARBs (losartan, valsartan, irbesartan, candesartan) do not cause cough.

When blood pressure cannot be adequately controlled with the maximum dose of an ACE inhibitor or ARB, additional antihypertensive medications may be needed, such as calcium channel blockers, alphablockers (indapamide) and centrally acting agents (clonidine patch). Patients with renal insufficiency and hypertension may be given a diuretic as part of the antihypertensive regimen because of related sodium and fluid retention; a loop diuretic usually is necessary if the creatinine level exceeds 2 mg/dL.

12

Protein intake should be limited to 0.8 g/kg/day or approximately 10% of daily calories, derived primarily from lean animal and vegetable or plant sources, in patients with diabetes and evidence of nephropathy. Vegetable proteins appear to have beneficial renal effects compared with animal sources and provide an important protein supplement or substitute in low-protein diets. The value of restricting protein intake in the absence of diabetic renal disease has not been clearly demonstrated. Low-protein diets can be made more palatable with a greater variety of vegetable protein sources and increased consumption of high-fiber complex carbohydrates and monounsaturated fats.

■ Diabetic Neuropathy

The various diabetic neuropathies are one of the most common yet distressing long-term complications of diabetes, affecting 60% to 70% of patients with type 1 and type 2 diabetes. The categories of diabetic neuropathy are shown in Table 12.9.

TABLE 12.9 — TYPES OF DIABETIC NEUROPATHIES
Sensorimotor Peripheral Neuropathies • Symmetric, distal, bilateral of upper/lower extremities • Mononeuropathies • Diabetic amyotrophy
Autonomic Neuropathies • Gastroparesis diabeticorum • Diabetic diarrhea • Neurogenic bladder • Impaired cardiovascular reflex responses • Impotence

Symmetric Distal Neuropathy

These neuropathies develop most often in the lower extremities, causing numbness and tingling (pins-and-needles paresthesias) usually during the night. Some patients develop painful burning and stabbing symptoms that can interfere with their quality of life and may be associated with neuropathic cachexia syndrome that includes anorexia, depression, and weight loss. Treatments that have varying degrees of effectiveness, particularly for painful neuropathies, include tricyclic antidepressants, carbamazepine, phenytoin, and counterirritants such as topical capsaicin. Aspirin or propoxyphene should be prescribed as necessary for pain; narcotic analgesics generally should be avoided because of the risk of addiction with chronic use, however, in some cases, these drugs are necessary. Gabapentin (Neurontin) and tramadol (Ultram) are newer medications that benefit a subset of patients with painful neuropathy.

In general, treatment strategies for painful peripheral neuropathy include initial use of nonsteroidal anti-inflammatory drugs, such as aspirin and Tylenol, which can offer pain relief, especially in patients with musculoskeletal or joint abnormalities secondary to long-standing neuropathy. The tricyclic antidepressants, such as amitriptyline, remain the most commonly used drugs in the treatment of painful neuropathy. After 6 weeks of treatment, many patients report significant pain relief, independent of mood but correlating with increasing drug dosage. The topical cream capsaicin may be added to the patient's therapeutic regimen if neuropathic pain persists in spite of treatment with maximally tolerated doses of antidepressant medication.

In an outpatient setting, approximately two thirds of diabetic patients treated with a combination of antidepressant medication and capsaicin cream experience substantial relief of neuropathic pain. In patients who experience continued pain on combination therapy, an anticonvulsant, such as gabapentin, or tramadol can be added as a third drug. If neuropathic pain persists despite the outlined treatment regimen, referral to a specialist, addition of a transcutaneous nerve stimulation (TENS) unit, acupuncture, or a series of local nerve blocks may be helpful, although the prognosis for pain relief in these patients is poor. A treatment flow chart for managing painful diabetic neuropathy is shown in Figure 12.3.

Mononeuropathy

These neuropathies can occur in virtually any cranial or peripheral nerve, are asymmetric, and have an abrupt onset. Cranial mononeuropathies are the most common, particularly the third and sixth, causing extraocular muscle motor paralysis and peripheral palsies. Patients can develop palsies involving the peroneal (foot drop), median, and ulner nerves. Spontaneous recovery over 3 to 6 months is typical. Patients with diabetes are more prone to developing compression neuropathies such as carpal tunnel syndrome.

Diabetic Amyotrophy

This neuropathy often is asymmetric, is more common in men, and is often characterized by severe pain, muscle wasting in the pelvic girdle and quadricep muscles, and mild sensory involvement. This condition usually is self-limiting, with complete recovery typically occurring in 6 to 12 months. Treatment is focused on maintaining glycemic control and symptomatic relief using physical therapy and analgesics.

Gastroparesis

This neuropathy should be suspected in patients with nausea, vomiting, early satiety, abdominal distention, and bloating following a meal, and is second-

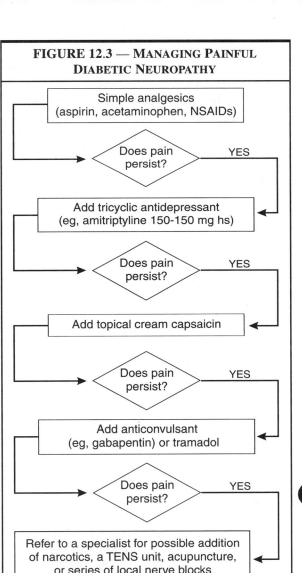

FIGURE 12.3 — MANAGING PAINFUL DIABETIC NEUROPATHY

Simple analgesics (aspirin, acetaminophen, NSAIDs)

Does pain persist? — YES

Add tricyclic antidepressant (eg, amitriptyline 150-150 mg hs)

Does pain persist? — YES

Add topical cream capsaicin

Does pain persist? — YES

Add anticonvulsant (eg, gabapentin) or tramadol

Does pain persist? — YES

Refer to a specialist for possible addition of narcotics, a TENS unit, acupuncture, or series of local nerve blocks

Abbreviations: NSAID, nonsteroidal anti-inflammatory drug; TENS, transcutaneous electrical nerve stimulation.

ary to delayed emptying and retention of gastric contents. The delay in gastric emptying usually is asymptomatic, although glycemic control can be affected. Postprandial hypoglycemia and delayed hyperglycemia develop when the balance between exogenous insulin administration and nutrient absorption is disrupted because of gastric stasis. Therefore, gastroparesis should be considered even in the absence of gastrointestinal symptoms in a patient who suddenly develops unexplainable poor glycemic control after having had satisfactory control.

Primary treatment is focused on optimizing glucose control with insulin; secondary treatment involves dietary modifications in the form of a low-fat, low-residue diet. When patients remain symptomatic despite these measures, treatment with the following prokinetic agents is recommended:

- Erythromycin lactobionate 1.5 to 3.0 mg/kg body weight IV every 6 to 8 hours (acute treatment, effective in eliminating residue from stomach); common side effects are nausea and vomiting.
- Oral treatment with cisapride (only obtained by special request because of cardiac side effects), 10 to 20 mg before meals and at bedtime (enhances gastric emptying through serotoninergic mechanisms, effective in acute conditions); minimal side effects (abdominal cramping, frequent bowel movements); long-term use may cause hyperprolactinemia, galactorrhea, menstrual irregularities.
- Oral metoclopramide HCl is generally used with caution because of adverse reactions (nervousness, anxiety, dystonic effects, and the potential for irreversible tardive dyskinesia).
- Oral treatment with domperidone, a peripheral dopamine antagonist (FDA approval pending), 10 to 20 mg 3 to 4 times daily (accelerates gas-

tric emptying); minimal side effects (abdominal cramping, frequent bowel movements) and rare adverse reactions (hyperprolactinemia, galactorrhea).

Diabetic Diarrhea

Intermittent diarrhea may alternate with constipation and can be difficult to treat. Diabetic diarrhea is a diagnosis of exclusion. High-fiber intake can be helpful, along with diphenoxylate (Lomotil), loperamide (Imodium), or clonidine. Small intestine stasis contributes to bacterial overgrowth, causing diarrhea. Treatment with one of the following antibiotics for 10 to 14 days is recommended:

- Doxycycline hyclate, 100 mg every 12 hours
- Amoxicillin trihydrate, 250 mg every 6 hours
- Metronidazole, 250 mg every 6 hours
- Ciprofloxacin HCl, 250 mg every 12 hours.

A trial of pancreatic enzymes is also recommended to rule out exocrine pancreatic insufficiency. In many instances, tincture of opium is the only medication that can help the patient live a nearly normal daily life.

Neurogenic Bladder

Frequent small voidings and incontinence that may progress to urinary retention characterize this neuropathy. Confirmation of this diagnosis requires demonstration of cystometric abnormalities and large residual urine volume. Most medical treatment is inadequate, although scheduling frequent voidings every 3 to 4 hours combined with bethanechol 10 to 50 mg 3 to 4 times daily supplemented by small doses of phenoxybenzamine may be helpful. Surgical intervention may be necessary if patients do not respond to pharmacologic therapy because chronic urinary retention can lead to urinary tract infection.

Impaired Cardiovascular Reflexes

Orthostatic hypotension and fixed tachycardia are the most disturbing and disabling autonomic symptoms. Typical treatment of orthostatic hypotension includes elevating the head of the bed, compression stockings for lower limbs and torso, supplementary salt intake, and the use of fludrocortisone (0.05 mg initially with gradual increases of 0.1 mg up to 0.5 to 1 mg). This pharmacologic therapy should be used cautiously in patients with cardiac disease because it causes sodium and water retention and may precipitate congestive heart failure.

Sexual Dysfunction

Erectile dysfunction, or impotence, is defined as the consistent inability for a man to get or keep an erection for satisfactory sexual intercourse. It is a couples' disorder, as both patient and partner suffer. Diabetic impotence is usually caused by circulatory and nervous system abnormalities and is a very common complaint in the male diabetic population. The classic clinical picture includes a patient with normal sexual desire but the inability to physically act on that desire. If a patient says that he has morning erections, he can masturbate without problems, or his libido is abnormally low, look for other causes of impotence such as psychological problems or a low androgen state. Orgasm and ejaculation are usually normal. Even if the patient does not have any psychological problems that could cause the impotence, he may develop a secondary psychological fear of failure that could complicate the clinical picture. A woman may experience lack of lubrication and painful intercourse.

The diagnosis can be made in most cases by a good sexual, psychosocial, and medical history, a physical examination, and laboratory tests. A testosterone level should be drawn to rule out a low androgen state, which is rarely a cause for impotence.

244

Hyperprolactinemia is also an uncommon cause of impotence. Hemochromatosis is a condition that is underdiagnosed and is associated with impotence and glucose intolerance. Serum iron stores, including ferritin levels, are abnormally high in this disorder. If the patient has femoral bruits and/or peripheral occlusive disease, then a vascular workup may help identify the cause of impotence.

It is important to be sure the patient is not taking any medications that can cause impotence such as β-blockers and thiazide diuretics. ACE inhibitors, ARBs, calcium-channel blockers, and α-blockers do not generally cause impotence.

Despite the prevalence of this disorder, nearly all patients can be successfully treated with either nonsurgical or surgical means. Yohimbine HCl, an α_2-adrenergic blocking agent, has been widely used as a nonhormonal medication for the treatment of impotence. However, there has been a consistent lack of data to show that it is more effective than placebo.

Testosterone given by injection or via a scrotal or skin patch is only indicated when the serum testosterone levels are low on several occasions. If there might be binding protein abnormalities, then a free testosterone level is indicated. As mentioned above, a low testosterone state is rarely a cause of impotence.

Sildenafil (Viagra), a selective inhibitor of phosphodiesterase type 5, inactivates cyclic GMP resulting in increase in nitric oxide levels. It has become the treatment of choice for most men with erectile dysfunction. A pilot study of 21 diabetic patients (types 1 and 2) with a mean age of 50 years examined the efficacy of sildenafil in doses up to 50 mg. Erectile function improvement was noted in 48% of the patients receiving 25 mg and 52% in patients receiving 50 mg.

The recommended dose of sildenafil is 25 mg, 50 mg, or 100 mg 1 hour before sexual activity. Following an initial starting dose of 50 mg, the dose may be increased or decreased based on efficacy and tolerability. Maximum dose is 100 mg. Side effects of the medication are headaches, light-headedness, dizziness, flushing, distorted vision, dyspepsia, syncope, and myocardial infarction.

Men at highest risk for syncope are those taking nitrates. It also has adverse effects in people with hypertrophic cardiomyopathy because a decrease in preload and afterload which can increase the outflow obstruction, culminating in an unstable hemodynamic state. The American College of Cardiology and the American Heart Association have published recommendations for the use of sildenafil. The document reiterates caution with respect to the use of sildenafil in the following situations:

- Patients with active coronary ischemia who are not taking nitrates
- Congestive heart failure and borderline blood pressure or low volume status
- Complicated, multidrug, antihypertensive regimen
- Patients taking drugs that prolong the half-life by blocking enzyme CYP3A4 (ie, erythromycin, cimetidine).

Vacuum constrictor devices are a viable therapeutic option for diabetic patients with impotence. No surgery or injections are required, patient acceptance is excellent, and there are few side effects. The majority of these external penile devices have a vacuum chamber that goes over the penis, a vacuum pump that creates negative pressure within the chamber allowing for engorgement of the penis with blood, and a constrictor band that is placed over the base of the penis when tumescence is achieved. Side effects are minor and include ecchymoses, hematomas, and pain. These devices are effective in men with both total and partial impotence. Many patients discover that they do not need the device after a brief period of time, which indicates that a fear of failure or other psychological problems were the initial cause of impotence.

Intracavernosal injection of vasoactive agents such as papaverine or prostaglandins can be self administered and work by relaxing corporal smooth muscle. Intracavernosal injections will work best in patients with diabetic impotence whose arterial inflow and corporal veno-occlusion mechanism is normal. Side effects include the formation of painless fibrotic nodules within the corpora cavernosa and priapism. Titration guidelines should be followed when initiating therapy. Despite the route of administration, patient acceptance is also good. Intraurethral (MUSE) are also available.

Penile prostheses represent an excellent surgical option for the treatment of impotence. The options range from simple malleable or semirigid prostheses to inflatable devices that use hydraulic principles to inflate and deflate the penis when desired. Surgical complications are very low, especially when the patient's glycemic control has been acceptable prior to surgery. With the availability of oral medications, intracavernosal injections, and vacuum devices, surgery is chosen less often.

Diabetic Foot Disorders

12

More than half of all nontraumatic amputations in the United States occur in individuals with diabetes, and the majority of these could have been prevented with proper foot care. Efforts aimed at prevention, early detection, and treatment of diabetic foot disorders can have a significant impact on the incidence of these problems.

■ Detection and Treatment

The physician and patient must diligently examine the feet on a regular basis for signs of redness or trauma, especially if neuropathy is present. Lack of pain, position, and vibratory sensations caused by neuropathy, associated deformities, and vascular ischemia can facilitate the development of foot lesions. Foot pressure that is abnormally distributed predisposes a neuropathic patient to pressure ischemia and skin breakdown. Autonomic neuropathy causes decreased sweating and dry skin that can result in cracked, thickened skin that is susceptible to infection and ulceration.

Pressure perception can be assessed using the Semmes Weinstein monofilaments, which are available in three thicknesses: 1-g fiber (SW 4.17 rating), 10-g fiber (SW 5.07 rating), and 75-g fiber (SW 6.10 rating). The following evaluation procedure has been recommended:

Place the monofilament against the skin and apply pressure to different areas of the bottom of the foot until the filament buckles. The patient should be able to feel the monofilament when it buckles and identify the location being tested. The 5.07 thickness monofilament, which is equivalent to 10-g of linear pressure, detects the presence or absence of protective sensation and is useful for identifying a foot at risk for ulceration and in need of special care.

Daily inspection of feet can help detect early skin lesions, and proper footwear can minimize the development of foot problems. Patients should be taught to cut toenails straight across and not trim calluses themselves, regularly wash their feet with warm water and mild soap, and avoid going barefoot or wearing constricting shoes. Minor wounds that are not infected can be treated with mild antiseptic solution, daily dressing changes, and foot rest. Patient guidelines for care of the diabetic foot are shown in Table 12.10.

Podiatrists should be consulted for assistance with more serious foot problems and for regular nail and callus care in high-risk individuals. If an ulcer develops, the skin must be debrided and the pressure alleviated; infections should be treated promptly with medications appropriate for the offending organism. Healing is facilitated by bed rest with foot elevation and the use of an orthopedic walking cast to relieve pressure but allow mobility. Intravenous antibiotics, surgical debridement, distal arterial revascularization, and local foot-sparing surgery may help prevent amputation in cases of seriously infected foot ulcers.

12

TABLE 12.10 — CARE OF THE DIABETIC FOOT

- Wash feet daily and dry carefully, especially between the toes. (Same after shower, jacuzzi, or swimming.)
- Inspect your feet daily for blisters, cuts, scratches, and areas of possible infection. Look between the toes! A mirror can help you see the bottom of your feet and between toes. If it is not possible for you to inspect your feet, seek the help of a family member or friend
- If your feet feel cold at night, wear socks. Do not apply hot water bottles or heating pads
- Avoid extreme temperatures for your feet. Test bath water with your hand to ensure that it is not too hot, and be extremely careful of hot pavement or concrete in the summer
- Inspect your shoes daily for foreign objects, nail points, torn linings, or other problems
- Change socks daily, wear properly fitting socks, and avoid holes or mended socks. "THOR-LO" socks have extra padding in heel and ball of foot for better shock absorption (available in sporting goods stores)
- All shoes should be comfortable at the time of purchase. Do not depend on shoes to break in. Wear them only 1 hour the first day, and only in the house. Check your feet for blisters, and then slowly increase the wearing time
- Do not wear sandals with thongs between the toes, and never wear shoes without socks
- Never walk barefoot, not even in the house, because of danger from stepping on pins, needles, tacks, glass, or other items on the floor
- Do not use chemical agents to remove corns or calluses, and do not cut them yourself; consult your podiatrist and be sure to let him/her know you are diabetic
- Toenails should be cut straight across. If you have trouble or questions about them, see your podiatrist.
- Infections from cuts, scratches, blisters, etc, can cause significant problems in diabetics, and a podiatrist or physician should be seen when infection occurs
- Do not smoke!

Goldman F, et al. In: *The High Risk Foot in Diabetes Mellitus*. New York, NY: Churchill Livingstone; 1990.

SUGGESTED READING

Abuaisha BB, Costanzi JB, Boulton AJ. Acupuncture for the treatment of chronic painful peripheral diabetic neuropathy: a long-term study. *Diabetes Res Clin Prac*. 1998;39:115-121.

American Diabetes Association. Clinical practice recommendations 2000. Preventive foot care in people with diabetes. *Diabetes Care*. 2000;23(suppl 1):S55-S56.

American Diabetes Association. *Diabetes 2002 Vital Statistics*. Alexandria, Va: American Diabetes Association; 2002.

Backonja M, Beydoun A, Edwards KR, et al. Gabapentin for the symptomatic treatment of painful neuropathy in patients with diabetes mellitus: a randomized controlled trial. *JAMA*. 1998;280: 1831-1836.

Brenner BM, Cooper ME, de Zeeuw D, et al. Effects of losartan on renal and cardiovascular outcomes in patients with type 2 diabetes and nephropathy. *N Engl J Med*. 2001:345:861-869.

Cheitlin MD, Hutter AM, Brindis RG, et al. Use of sildenafil (Viagra) in patients with cardiovascular disease. Technology and Practice Executive Committee. *Circulation*. 1999;99:168-177.

Cohen KL, Harris S. Efficacy and safety of nonsteroidal anti-inflammatory drugs in the therapy of diabetic neuropathy. *Arch Intern Med*. 1987;147:1442-1444.

Davidson MB. *Diabetes Mellitus*: *Diagnosis and Treatment*, 3rd ed. New York, NY: Churchill Livingstone; 1991.

Diabetes Control and Complications Trial Research Group. The effect of intensive treatment of diabetes on the development and progression of long-term complications in insulin-dependent diabetes mellitus. *N Engl J Med*. 1993; 329:977-986.

Diabetic Retinopathy Study Research Group. Indications for photocoagulation treatment of diabetic retinopathy, DRS report no. 14. *Int Ophthalmol Clin*. 1987;27:239-253.

Early Treatment Diabetic Retinopathy Study Research Group. Photocoagulation for diabetic macular edema: ETDRS report no. 1. *Ophthalmology*. 1985;103;1796-1806.

12

Edelman SV, White D, Henry RR. Intensive insulin therapy for patients with type II diabetes. *Curr Opin Endocrinol Diab.* 1995;2:333-340.

Goldman F, Gibbons G, Kruse-Edelmann I. Limb salvage techniques. In: *The High Risk Foot in Diabetes Mellitus.* New York, NY: Churchill Livingstone; 1990.

Gorson KC, Schott C, Herman R, Ropper AH, Rand WM. Gabapentin in the treatment of painful diabetic neuropathy: a placebo controlled, double blind, crossover trial. *J Neurol Neurosurg Psychiatry.* 1999;66:251-252.

Harati Y, Gooch C, Swenson M, et al. Double-blind randomized trial of tramadol for the treatment of the pain of diabetic neuropathy. *Neurology.* 1998;50:1842-1846.

Heart Outcomes Prevention Evaluation (HOPE) Study Investigators. Effects of ramipril on cardiovascular and microvascular outcomes in people with diabetes mellitus: results of the HOPE study and MICRO-HOPE substudy. *Lancet.* 2000;355:253-259.

Isomaa B, Almgren P, Tuomi T, et al. Cardiovascular morbidity and mortality associated with the metabolic syndrome. *Diabetes Care.* 2001;24:683-689.

Karlsson FO, Garber AJ. Prevention and treatment of diabetic nephropathy: role of angiotensin-converting enzyme inhibitors. *Endocr Pract.* 1996;2:215-219.

Krowlewski AS, Laffel LM, Krolewski M, Quinn M, Warram JH. Glycosylated hemoglobin and the risk of microalbuminuria in patients with insulin-dependent diabetes mellitus. *N Engl J Med.* 1995;332:1251-1255.

Kumar D, Marshall HJ. Diabetic peripheral neuropathy: amelioration of pain with transcutaneous electrostimulation. *Diabetes Care.* 1997;20:1702-1705.

Labasky RC, Spivack AP. Transurethral alprostadil for treatment of erectile dysfunction: Two-year safety update. *J Urol.* 1998;159:907A.

Lakin MM, Montague DK, Vander Brug Medendorp S, Tesar L, Schover LR. Intracavernous injection therapy: analysis of results and complications. *J Urol.* 1990;143:1138-1141.

Leungwattanakij S, Flynn V, Hellstrom WJ. Intracavernosal injection and intraurethral therapy for erectile dysfunction. *Urol Clin North Am*. 2001;28:343-354.

Levine LA, Dimitiou RJ. Vacuum constriction and external erection devices in erectile dysfunction. *Urol Clin North Am*. 2001;28: 355-361.

Lewis E, Hunsicker LG, Bain RP, Rohde RD. The effect of angiotensin-converting enzyme inhibition on diabetic nephropathy. *N Engl J Med*. 1993;329:1456-1462.

Lewis EJ, Hunsicker LG, Clarke WR, et al. Renoprotective effect of the angiotensin-receptor antagonist irbesartan in patients with nephropathy due to type 2 diabetes. *N Engl J Med*. 2001:345:851-860.

Max MB, Culnane M, Schafer SC, et al. Amitriptyline relieves diabetic neuropathy pain in patients with normal or depressed mood. *Neurology*. 1987;37:589-596.

McQuay HJ, Tramer M, Nye BA, Carroll D, Wiffen PJ, Moore RA. A systematic review of antidepressants in neuropathic pain. *Pain*. 1996;68:217-227.

Montague DK, Angermeier KW. Penile prosthesis implantation. *Urol Clin North Am*. 2001;28:355-361.

Mudaliar SR, Henry RR. Role of glycemic control and protein restriction in clinical management of diabetic kidney disease. *Endocrinol Pract*. 1996;2:220-226.

Padma-Nathan H, Giuliano F. Oral drug therapy for erectile dysfunction. *Urol Clin North Am*. 2001;28:321-334.

Parving HH, Lehnert H, Brochner-Mortensen J, Gomis R, Andersen S, Arner P. The effect of irbesartan on the development of diabetic nephropathy in patients with type 2 diabetes. *N Engl J Med*. 2001:345:870-878.

Peragallo-Dittko V, ed. *A Core Curriculum for Diabetes Education*, 2nd ed. Chicago, Ill: American Association of Diabetes Educators; 1993.

Prather CM. Evaluating and managing GI dysfunction in diabetes. *Contemp Intern Med*. 1996;8:47-54.

12

Reichard P, Nilsson BY, Rosenqvist U. The effect of long-term intensified insulin treatment on the development of microvascular complications of diabetes mellitus. *N Engl J Med*. 1993;329:304-309.

Rendell MS, Rajfer J, Wicker PA, Smith MD. Sildenafil for the treatment of erectile dysfunction in men with diabetes: randomized controlled trial. Sildenafil Diabetes Study Group. *JAMA*. 1999;281:421-426.

United Kingdom Prospective Diabetes Study Group. Efficacy of atenolol and captopril in reducing risk of macrovascular and microvascular complications in type 2 diabetes: UKPDS 39. *BMJ*. 1998;317:713-720.

United Kingdom Prospective Diabetes Study. VIII. Study design, progress, and performance. *Diabetologia*. 1991;34:877-890.

13 Resources

American Association of Diabetes Educators (AADE)
444 N. Michigan Avenue, Suite 1240
Chicago, IL 60611
312/644-2233 or 800/338-3633
800/TEAMUP4 (800/832-6874) (Diabetes Educator Access Line)
Website: www.diabetesnet.com/aade.html

AADE is a multidisciplinary organization, with state and regional chapters, for health professionals involved in diabetes patient education. The organization sponsors a certification program for diabetes educators and provides grants, scholarships, and awards for educational research and teaching activities. AADE's annual meeting features continuing education programs on diabetes treatment and education. The organization also features a Diabetes Educator Access Line to help people with diabetes locate diabetes education services in their area.

Publications: AADE publishes a bimonthly journal, *The Diabetes Educator*; curriculum guides; consensus statements; self-study programs; and other print and nonprint resources for diabetes educators.

American Diabetes Association (ADA)
ADA National Service Center
1660 Duke Street
Alexandria, VA 22314
703/549-1500 or 800/342-2383
Website: www.diabetes.org

ADA is both a professional association and a private, nonprofit, voluntary organization with state and local affiliates and chapters. It serves people with diabetes and their families and friends, as well as health professionals and research scientists involved in diabetes-related activities. The organization funds diabetes research and education activities; sponsors educational programs, including an annual meeting, postgraduate courses, consensus meetings, and special symposia; administers a recognition program for diabetes outpatient education; develops professional guidelines for diabetes care; and advocates for diabetes issues in the legislative and public health arenas. Local ADA affiliates often sponsor educational programs and support groups for persons with diabetes and their families.

Publications: ADA publishes monthly and quarterly magazines for patients, including *Diabetes Forecast*; professional journals focusing on basic and clinical research, including *Diabetes, Diabetes Care, Diabetes Spectrum,* and *Diabetes Reviews*; other publications, including cookbooks, meal planing guides, pamphlets, brochures, and books for patients; and clinical manuals, nutritional guides, audiovisuals, statistical reports, and curriculum guides for professionals.

Division of Diabetes Translation
National Center for Chronic Disease Prevention
and Health Promotion
Centers for Disease Control and Prevention (CDC)
Mail Stop K-10
4770 Buford Highway NE
Atlanta, GA 30341-3717
770/488-5000
Website: www.cdc.gov/diabetes

An agency of the Public Health Service, Department of Health and Human Services, CDC develops public health approaches to reduce the burden of diabetes in the United States. The agency supports diabetes control programs in 26 states and one territory; carries out state and national surveillance activities to assess diabetes prevalence, impact, and possible contributing factors; develops consensus guidelines for clinical and public health practice; supports community-based preventive programs for minority populations and the elderly; and coordinates Federal activities concerned with translating research findings into clinical practice, including issues related to cost and reimbursement practices, disability, and quality of life.

Publications: CDC distributes a practice manual for primary-care practitioners and a companion guide for patients, surveillance reports, and guidelines on patient education, educational reimbursement, and maternal and child health. State programs have produced patient and professional publications.

Indian Health Services (IHS)
IHS Headquarters West
Central Diabetes Program
5300 Homestead Road NE
Albuquerque, NM 87110
505/248-4182
www.ihs.gov

An agency of the Public Health Service, Department of Health and Human Services, IHS supports 17 model Diabetes Health Care Programs serving Native Americans and Alaskans. These programs develop and evaluate effective and culturally accepted prevention and treatment methods for diabetes and its complications. Diabetes control officers in each IHS region provide surveillance, training, and other services to promote the use of techniques recommended by the program.

Publications: The model programs and the IHS produce culturally relevant publications for native populations, including nutrition guides, complication-specific educational materials, and guides for professionals. Publications are available only to persons working with Native Americans or Alaskan populations.

International Diabetes Center (IDC)
3800 Park Nicollet Boulevard
Minneapolis, MN 55416
888/825-6315 or 952/993-3393
Website: www.idcdiabetes.org

A division of the Park Nicollet Medical Foundation, IDC offers education classes for people with diabetes and training programs for health professionals. The programs for health professionals focus on team management of diabetes. IDC also provides inpatient and outpatient treatment services in adult and pediatric clinics, supports clinical research to assess new diabetes care systems and approaches, conducts psychosocial research, and supports a network of IDC satellite centers that offer specialized programs in diabetes. The IDC has been designated as a World Health Organization Collaborating Center for Diabetes Education and Training.

13

Publications: The organization publishes *Living Well with Diabetes*, a quarterly magazine for people with diabetes. Other publications include management and nutrition guides for patients, low-literacy patient education booklets, guides for health professionals, audiovisuals, and general publications related to chronic health problems and nutrition. For publications/mail order pharmacy services: Chronimed; PO Box 47945; Minneapolis, MN 55447-9727; 800/876-6540 or 612/546-1146.

International Diabetes Federation (IDF)
1 Rue DeFacqz
1000 Brussels, Belgium
322/538-5511
www.idf.org

IDF collaborates with more than 100 member associations in over 80 countries, the World Health Organization, and other affiliated organizations and individuals to ensure that people with diabetes receive quality treatment and education services.

Publications: IDF publishes a newsletter, a journal entitled *IDF Bulletin, The Directory 1991: A Guide to the Activities of Member Diabetes Associations*, as well as other publications.

Joslin Diabetes Center
One Joslin Place
Boston, MA 02215
617/732-2400 or 800/JOSLIN-1 (800/567-5461)
Website: www.joslin.org

The Joslin Diabetes Center offers inpatient and outpatient treatment, education, and other support services to adults and children with diabetes; provides professional medical education; sponsors camps for children with diabetes; and supports research to improve treatment and find a cure for diabetes and its complications. The center is affiliated with Harvard Medical School and a number of hospitals in the Boston area and operates affiliated clinics in several states. The Joslin Diabetes Center is one of six Diabetes Endocrinology Research Centers supported by the National Institute of Diabetes and Digestive Kidney Diseases.

Publications: Joslin produces a variety of educational materials for patients and professionals, including manuals, nutrition guides, materials for children with diabetes, and films. *The Joslin Magazine* is issued quarterly to members of the Joslin Society.

Juvenile Diabetes Foundation (JDF) International
120 Wall Street, 19th Floor
New York, NY 10005-4001
212/785-9595 or 800/JDF-CURE (800/533-2873)
Website: www.jdfcure.org

JDF is a private, nonprofit, voluntary organization with chapters throughout the world. JDF raises funds to support research on the cause, cure, treatment, and prevention of diabetes and its complications. The organization awards research grants for laboratory and clinical investigations and sponsors a variety of career development and research training programs for new and established investigators. JDF also sponsors international workshops and conferences for biomedical researchers. Individual chapters offer support groups and other activities for families.

Publications: JDF publishes the quarterly journal *Countdown* and a series of patient education brochures about insulin-dependent and non–insulin-dependent diabetes.

Mayo Clinic Health Oasis
Mayo Foundation for Medical Education and Research
200 First Street SW
Rochester, MN 55905
507/284-2511
Website: www.mayohealth.org

This site is directed by a team of Mayo Clinic physicians, scientists, writers and educators. IT is updated each weekday. This website has reliable information for a healthier life about many topics, including diabetes. Diabetes information includes links to other websites, emergencies, long-term complications, drug updates, prevention, treatments, transplantations, etc.

National Diabetes Education Initiative (NDEI)
A division of Physicians World Communications Group
400 Plaza Drive
Secaucus, NJ 07094
201/865-7500 or 800/223-8978
Website: www.ndei.org

13

The NDEI is a multicomponent educational program on type 2 diabetes that is designed for endocrinologists, diabetologists, primary-care physicians, and other health-care professionals. NDEI programs address issues such as epidemiology and pathophysiology, rational for treatment and management guidelines, microvascular and macrovascular complications, therapeutic options and prevention.

National Diabetes Education Program (NDEP)
c/o National Diabetes Information Clearinghouse (NDIC)
1 Information Way
Bethesda, MD 20892-3560
800/860-8747 or 301/654-3327
website: http://niddk.nih.gov/health/diabetes/diabetes.htm

NDEP is a federally sponsored initiative that involves public and private partners to improve the treatment and outcomes for people with diabetes, to promote early diagnosis and ultimately to prevent the onset of diabetes. NDEP is sponsored by the National Institute of Diabetes and Digestive and Kidney Disease (NIDDK) of the National Institutes of Health (NIH) and the Division of Diabetes Translation of the Centers for Disease Control and Prevention (CDC).

Publications: NDEP offers a variety of publications and videos for use by the general public, people with diabetes, and healthcare providers. These materials are provided in both English and Spanish formats.

National Eye Institute (NEI)
National Eye Health Education Program
2020 Vision Place
Bethesda, MD 20892-3655
301/496-5248 or 800/869-2020
Website: www.nei.nih.gov

NEI, one of the National Institutes of Health, supports basic and clinical research to develop effective treatments for diabetic eye disease. The institute's National Eye Health Education Program promotes public and professional awareness of the importance of early diagnosis and treatment of diabetic eye disease.

Publications: NEI produces patient and professional education materials related to diabetic eye disease and its treatment, including literature for patients, guides for health professionals, and education kits for community health workers and for pharmacists.

National Health Council
Suite 500
1730 M Street NW
Washington, DC 20036
202/785-3910
Website: www.nhcouncil.org

The National Health Council is a private, nonprofit umbrella organization comprised of more than 100 national health-related organizations, including over 40 of the nation's leading patient-based groups, also known as voluntary health agencies. The mission is to promote the health of all people by advancing the voluntary health movement.

National Institute of Diabetes and Digestive and Kidney Diseases (NIDDK)
National Institutes of Health (NIH)
31 Center Drive, MSC 2560
Bethesda, MD 20892-2560
301/496-4000
Website: www.niddk.nih.gov

The NIDDK conducts and supports research on many of the most serious diseases affecting public health, including diabetes. The website has information about the NIDDK, news releases, event information, health information and education programs, patient recruitment, coordination of federal programs, and research funding and programs.

National Kidney Foundation
Suite 1100
30 East 33rd St.
New York, NY 10016
212/889-2210 or 800/622-9010
Website: www.kidney.org

The National Kidney Foundation is a major voluntary health organization, seeking to prevent kidney and urinary tract diseases, improve the health and well-being of individuals and families affected by these diseases, and increase the availability of all organs for transplantation. The website has information for organ and tissue donors and recipients, health care professionals, patients, meetings and events.

13

National Stroke Association (NSA)
9707 E. Easter Lane
Englewood, CO 80112
303/649-9299 or 800/STROKES (800/787-6537)
Website: www.stroke.org

> The National Stroke Association's mission is to reduce the incidence and impact of stroke by changing the way stroke is viewed and treated. NSA is the only national organization dedicating 100% of its resources and efforts toward stroke through prevention, treatment, rehabilitation, research and support for stroke survivors and their families.

Taking Control of Your Diabetes
1110 Camino Del Mar, Suite B
Del Mar, CA 92014
800/99-TCOYD (800/998-2693)
or 858/755-5683 (main line)
858/755-6854 (fax)
website: www.tcoyd.org

> *Taking Control of Your Diabetes* (TCOYD) is a nonprofit organization dedicated to promoting advocacy programs for people with diabetes. The two main goals of the organization are to (1) educate people with diabetes about how to live longer by learning about their condition, and (2) educate patients to be self-advocates and work within their health care program to get the help they need to maintain a high standard of care. TCOYD maintains their mission by producing large patient-oriented educational and motivational events nationwide, in addition to providing educational videos, audio tapes, and reading materials. TCOYD also conducts a series of medical education seminars for professionals. TCOYD has an 800 number help line and website to assist people with diabetes and their families.

INDEX

Note: Page numbers in *italics* indicate figures;
page numbers followed by t refer to tables.

Abdominal obesity, definition of, 48t-49t
Acanthosis nigricans
  diabetes secondary to, 31t
  in dysmetabolic syndrome, 49t
Acarbose (Precose), 79. See also *α-glucosidase inhibitors.*
  in combination therapy, 98
  in diabetes type 2 prevention, 78
  dosage of, 84t, 98
  effectiveness of, 98
  patient instructions for, 100t
  for patients with acceptable fasting glucose but elevated
      glycohemoglobin, 112
  pharmacokinetics of, 98
  repaglinide interaction with, 106
  side effects of, 99
Accu-Chek blood glucose monitors, 166t, 170t
ACE inhibitors. See *Angiotensin-converting enzyme (ACE) inhibitors.*
Acesulfame K, 62
Acetohexamide (Dymelor), 82t, 101. See also *Sulfonylureas.*
Acidosis. See also *Ketoacidosis.*
  lactic, 96
  metabolic, 193
  renal tubular, 217
Acromegaly, 31t
Actos. See *Pioglitazone.*
ADA. See *American Diabetes Association.*
Adipose tissue. See also *Body fat distribution and type 2 diabetes.*
  insulin resistance in, 70-71
  PPARs in, 81
Adolescents, body weight of, type 2 diabetes risk and, 36-37
Adrenergic blockers. See *α-blockers; β-blockers.*
African Americans and type 2 diabetes
  diagnosis of, 39
  prevalence of, 11, 15, 32, 77
Age/aging. See also *Elderly people.*
  diabetes classification and, 30t-31t
  ideal body weight and, 55t
    type 2 diabetes risk and, 36-37
  impaired glucose tolerance progression and, 35
  malnutrition-related diabetes and, 34
  type 2 diabetes and, 20
    pathophysiologic sequence in, 20-21
    prevalence of, 11, *12*, 33
Alanine aminotransferase, in ketoacidosis, 195t
Alcohol intake
  blood glucose and, 63
  chlorpropamide and, 102
  false glycated hemoglobin reading and, 158
  insulin therapy and, 64
  nutrition therapy and, 58t-59t, 63
Aldosteronism, 31t

14

α-Blockers, 237, 245
  potential benefits of, 216t, 218
  side effects of, 215t
α-Glucosidase inhibitors
  dosage of, 84t
  indications for, *152-153*
  for obese type 2 diabetes patients with/without dyslipidemia, 111
  for patients with acceptable fasting glucose but elevated
    glycohemoglobin, 112
  pharmacokinetics of, 84t, 97-99, 100t
  for thin elderly patients, 112
Amaryl (glimepiride). See also *Sulfonylureas.*
  availability of, 102
  dosage and pharmacokinetics of, 82t, 104
American Association of Diabetes Education (AADE), 255
American Diabetes Association (ADA)
  address of, 255
  criteria of
    for diabetes diagnosis, 34t, 41t
    for impaired glucose tolerance, 34t
  dyslipidemia treatment priority of, 222t, 225t
  glycemic guidelines of, 73t, 150t
American Indians. See *Native Americans.*
Amitriptyline, 240
Amoxicillin trihydrate, 243
Amylase, in ketoacidosis, 195t
Amylin analog, 116
Amyotrophy, 240
Analgesics, nephropathy and, 234
Anemia, false glycated hemoglobin reading and, 158
Angiotensin-converting enzyme (ACE) inhibitors
  cardioprotective effects of, 214, 216t, 217
  for dysmetabolic syndrome, 47
  potassium restriction with, 63, 217
  renal effects of, 216t
  serum potassium and, 217
  side effects of, 215t
  stroke and, 216t
Angiotensin II receptor blockers (ARBs)
  CALM study of, 217
  for dysmetabolic syndrome, 47
  indications for, 237
  potential benefits of, 216t
  side effects of, 215t
Anti-rejection drugs, 122, 146-147
Anticonvulsants, for neuropathy, 240
Antidepressants, for neuropathy, 239
Antidiabetic agents, oral. See also specific agent.
  availability of, 79
  characteristics of, 82t-84t
  combination therapy with, 79-80, 114-115, *153.* See also *Insulin
    therapy, combined with oral agents.*
  contraindications for, 80
  under development, 116-117
  with diet and exercise, 79
  duration of use of, 79
  failure of, 79
  for glucose toxicity, 113
  indications for, *152*

264

Antidiabetic agents, oral *(continued)*
    for lean type 2 diabetes, 113
    monotherapy with, 111
    for obese type 2 diabetes patients with/without dyslipidemia, 111
    for patients with acceptable fasting glucose but elevated
        glycohemoglobin, 112
    for thin elderly patients, 112
    in treatment algorithm, *152*
Antihypertensive agents
    diabetes secondary to, 31t
    for diabetic nephropathy, 237
    guidelines for, 214
    potential benefits of, 216t
    side effects of, 215t
Antioxidant supplementation, 63
ARBs. See *Angiotensin receptor blockers.*
Asian Americans and type 2 diabetes, 11, 122
Asian Indians, type 2 diabetes in, 11, 15, 77
Aspart (Novolog)
    advantages of, 124
    effectiveness of, *123*, 138, 141
    indications for, 124-125
    pharmacokinetics of, *123*
    switching to glargine from, 142-143
Aspartame, 62
Aspartate aminotransferase, in ketoacidosis, 195t
Aspirin. See also *Nonsteroidal anti-inflammatory drugs.*
    for dysmetabolic syndrome, 48
    false glycated hemoglobin reading and, 159
    for neuropathy, 240
Assure blood glucose monitors, 166t, 170t
Atenolol, in UKPDS, 217-218
Atherosclerosis
    diet and, 63
    hypertension and, 213
AtLast glucose monitor, 166t, 170t
Atorvastatin (Lipitor), 224, 228
Avandia. See *Rosiglitazone.*

Basel insulins, 126t
Bedtime glucose level, ADA guidelines for, 73t, 150t
Behavior modification, in nutrition therapy, 54
Benzothiazepines, 218
β-Blockers, 31t
    contraindications for, 218
    potential benefits of, 216t, 218
    side effects of, 215t, 245
Beta cells
    in diabetes natural history, 22
    exhaustion of, 79
        insulin therapy for, 121
        sulfonylurea-induced, 104
    normal functioning of, 20
Bicarbonate therapy
    in HHNS, 203
    in hyperkalemia, 198
    in ketoacidosis, 198
Biguanide, 83t
Bile acid-binding resins, lipoprotein levels and, 226t

14

Bile acid sequestrants, 224, 227
Bladder, neurogenic, 243
  nephropathy and, 234
Bleeding, false glycated hemoglobin reading and, 158
Blood pressure. See also *Hypertension.*
  in diabetes warranty program, *44*
  in dysmetabolic syndrome, 48t
  therapeutic goals for, 156t
Blood urea nitrogen, in ketoacidosis, 194t
Body build, ideal body weight and, 56
Body fat distribution and type 2 diabetes. See also *Adipose tissue.*
  diagnosis and, 39
  etiologic sequence and, 22
  impaired glucose tolerance progression to, 35
Body weight. See also *Body fat distribution; Obesity; Weight gain; Weight loss.*
  in adolescents and children, type 2 diabetes risk and, 36-37
  in diabetes warranty program, *44*
  ideal, 55t, 56
  macrovascular risk and, 213
  in nutrition therapy goals, 53

C-peptide level, for insulin therapy combined with oral agents, 131
Calcium channel blockers, 237
  potential benefits of, 216t
  side effects of, 215t
  subclasses of, 218
Calorie intake
  distribution of, 54
  for weight loss, 56, 223, 224t
Cancer, death from, *17*
Candesartan, 237
Candesartan and Lisinopril Microalbuminuria (CALM) study, 217
Capsaicin, topical, 239
Captopril, in UKPDS, 217-218
Carbamazepine, 239
Carbohydrate intake
  carbohydrate complexity and, 97-98
  distribution of, 54
  recommended daily allowance of, 60
  sources of, 60-61
Carbohydrate replacement, for hypoglycemia, 205
Carbuncles, 208t
Cardiologist, in diabetes warranty program, *45*
Cardiovascular disorders. See also *Macrovascular disorders; Microvascular disorders.*
  ACE inhibitors and, 214, 217
  death from, *17*
  dyslipidemia and, 220
    nutrition and drug therapy for, 222t, 225t-226t
  fat intake and, 59-60, 220, 223, 224t
  fludrocortisone in, 244
  glitazones and, 81
  in HHNS, 203
  postprandial hyperglycemia and, 71
  risk assessment for, 43, 46-47
  in type 2 diabetes, 69, 244
CARE (Cholesterol and Recurrent Events), 226t
Carpal tunnel syndrome, 240

Cataracts, diet and, 63
Catecholamines, 31t
Cellulitis, 209t
Centers for Disease Control and Prevention (CDC), 256
Cerebrovascular disorders, death from, *17*
Cerivastatin, 224
CheckMate Plus, 166t, 171t
Children, body weight of, type 2 diabetes risk and, 36-37
Chlorpropamide (Diabinese). See also *Sulfonylureas.*
    alcohol intake and, 102
    availability of, 101
    dosage and pharmacokinetics of, 82t
    side effects of, 102
Cholesterol and Recurrent Events (CARE), 226t
Cholesterol intake, 60, 223
Cholesterol level
    acceptable, 221t
    calculation of, 220
Cholestid, 224
Ciprofloxacin, 243
Cisapride, 242
Classification of diabetes mellitus, 29-37. See also specific category, eg,
    Gestational diabetes mellitus.
    distinguishing characteristics in, 30t-31t
    problems in, 36-37
Clonidine patch, 237
Coexisting medical conditions
    in pathophysiology of type 2 diabetes, 22
    pharmacologic therapy and, 69-70
    in progression of impaired glucose tolerance to type 2 diabetes, 35
Cognitive impairment
    in HHNS, 202
    in type 2 diabetes, 210
Complications of insulin therapy
    hypoglycemia as, 145-146
    weight gain as, 145
Complications of type 2 diabetes. See also specific complication,
    eg, *Retinopathy.*
    acute, 189-210
    cardiovascular reflex impairment as, 244
    death from, *17*
    diarrhea as, 243
    dyslipidemia as, 219-228
    foot disorders as, 247-249, 250t
    HHNS as, 198-199, 200t-201t, 202-203
    hypertension as, 213-219
    hypoglycemia as, 203-207
    infection as, 39, 207, 208t-209t
    ketoacidosis as. See *Ketoacidosis.*
    long-term, 211-249, 250t
    macrovascular, 212-219
    metabolic, 189-207
    microvascular, 228-247
    nephropathic, 233-238
    neurogenic bladder as, 234, 243
    neuropathy as, 238-242
    retinopathy as, 228-233
    sexual dysfunction as, 244-247
Congestive heart failure, 244

14

Continuous subcutaneous insulin infusion, 128t
Coronary heart disease
    dyslipidemia and, nutrition and drug therapy for, 222t, 225t-226t
    in dysmetabolic syndrome, 49t
Cranial mononeuropathy, 240
Creatine
    in ketoacidosis, 194t
    in serum and clearance of, in diabetes warranty program, *45*
Creatinine phosphokinase level, lipid-lowering drugs and, 227
Cushing's syndrome, 31t
Cutaneous infections, 208t
Cystic fibrosis, 31t

DCCT. See *Diabetes Control and Complications Trial (DCCT)*
    recommendations.
Death from diabetes, 16, *17*
Dehydration, ketoacidosis and, 190
Dental examination, in diabetes warranty program, *44*
Dextrose
    for HHNS, 203
    for hypoglycemia, 206
DiaBeta. See *Glyburide.*
Diabetes Control and Complications Trial (DCCT) recommendations
    for intensive therapy, 151, 211-212
    for microvascular complication prevention, 211
    for nephropathy management, 236
    for SMBG, 162
    UKPDS results similarity to, 73, 74t
Diabetes mellitus, death from, *17*
Diabetes mellitus type 1
    distinguishing characteristics of, 29, 30t, 32
    late-onset, 113
    onset age in, 32
    prevalence of, 32
Diabetes mellitus type 2
    age and, 20
    death in, *17*
    distinguishing characteristics of, 30t, 32
    early intervention in, 24-25
    GDM progression to, 36-37
    hypertension and, 156t
    impaired glucose tolerance progression to, 35
    lean
        combined insulin and oral agent therapy for, 131
        oral antidiabetic agents for, 112
        predominant defect in, 70-71
    metabolic defects in, 22
    preventing or delaying onset of, 78
    in TRIPOD study, 78
    undiagnosed, 11, 13, 33
Diabetes Prevention Program (DPP)
    structure and results of, 77
    type 2 diabetes risk factors in, 76-77
Diabetes warranty program, 43, *44-*
Diabetic ketoacidosis. See *Ketoacidosis.*
Diabinese. See *Chlorpropamide.*
Diagnosis of diabetes
    ADA criteria for, 34t, 41t
    age at, 32

Diagnosis of diabetes *(continued)*
  asymptomatic, 39
  fasting glucose in, 35, 41t
  oral glucose tolerance testing in, 34t
  risk factors in, 39-40
  in routine physical examination, 39
  symptoms in, 33, 39
  in treatment algorithm, *152-153*
  type 1 vs type 2, 32
Dialysis, prognosis of, 234-235
Diarrhea, diabetic, 243
Diet. See *Nutrition therapy.*
Dietitian consult, 52-53
Dihydropyridines, 218
Diphenoxylate (Lomotil), 243
Diuretics
  diabetes secondary to, 31t
  indications for, 237
  insulin secretion and, 163
  potassium supplementation with, 63
  potential benefits of, 216t, 219
  side effects of, 215t, 245
Division of Diabetes Translation, National Center for Chronic Disease
    Prevention and Health Promotion, Centers for Disease Control and
    Prevention (CDC), 256
Domperidone, 242
DPP. See *Diabetes Prevention Program.*
Drug therapy. See *Antidiabetic agents, oral; Pharmacologic therapy;*
    specific drug or drug type.
Duet Glucose Control Monitor, 167t, 171t
Dymelor (acetohexamide), 82t, 101. See also *Sulfonylureas.*
Dyslipidemia. See also *Lipoprotein level.*
  ADA treatment priority in, 222t, 225t
  diet therapy for, 223, 224t
  drugs for, 224, 227
  fat intake and, 59, 220, 223, 224t
  in type 2 diabetes, 76, 219-220, 221t, 223-224, 224t-226t, 227-228
Dysmetabolic syndrome
  components of, 43, 46-47
  criteria for, 48t-49t
  treatment of, 47-49
Ear infection, 209t
Early Treatment Diabetic Retinopathy Study (ETDRS), 232
Edema, macular, 229, 233t
Elderly people. See also *Age/aging.*
  anti-glutamic acid decarboxylase antibodies in, 139
  HHNS in, 198
  hypoglycemia in, 163
  insulin pump therapy in, 139
  ketoacidosis in, 191
  quality of life of, 210
  sulfonylurea-induced hypoglycemia in, 103
  thin, oral antidiabetic agents for, 112
Electrolyte depletion, in ketoacidosis, 190, 196
Endocrinopathies, diabetes secondary to, 31t
Epinephrine production, ketoacidosis and, 190
Erectile dysfunction
  definition of, 244
  diagnosis of, 244

14

269

Erectile dysfunction *(continued)*
  drug-induced, 245
  hemochromatosis and, 245
  hyperprolactinemia and, 240
  pathophysiology of, 244
  psychological issues in, 244
  treatment of, 245-247
Erythromycin lactobionate, 242
Estrogen-containing agents, 31t
Ethnicity and type 2 diabetes. See *Race/ethnicity and type 2 diabetes.*
ExacTech blood glucose monitors, 167t, 171t
Exercise. See also *Sedentary lifestyle.*
  aerobic, 66
  benefits of, 65
  duration and intensity of, 68t
  for dysmetabolic syndrome, 47
  guidelines for, 67t
  in hypertension treatment, 213
  hypoglycemia in, 66
  macrovascular risk and, 213
  nutrition therapy with, 53, 58t
  pharmacologic therapy and, 66, 79
  precautions before, 65-66
  prescription for, 66-67, 68t
  SMBG before and after, 66
  timing of, 207
  in treatment algorithm, *152*
Extend Bar, 207
Extendin-4, 117
Eye examination, in diabetes warranty program, *45*

Fat intake
  hyperlipidemia and, 59, 220, 223, 224t
  in nutrition therapy, 58t
  recommended daily allowance of, 60
  in weight loss programs, 60
Fat substitutes, 62
Fenofibrate (Tricor), 227
Fetal hemoglobin, false glycated hemoglobin reading and, 158
Fetus, GDM effects on, 36
Fibric acid derivatives, lipoprotein levels and, 226t
FK 506, 147
Fludrocortisone, 244
Fluid replacement therapy, in ketoacidosis, 193, 196-197
Fluvastatin, 224
Foot
  care of, 250t
  disorders of, 247-249
  examination of, in diabetes warranty program, *44*
Foot drop, 240
4S (Scandinavian Simvastatin Survival Study), 226t
FreeStyle glucose monitor, 167t, 171t
Fructosamine level, 159-160, *161*
Fructose intake, 61
Fruit intake, 61
Furunculosis, 208t

Gabapentin (Neurontin), 239-240

Gastric emptying
   in gastroparesis, 240-241
   postprandial hyperglycemia and, 71-72
Gastrointestinal disorders, in HHNS, 199
Gastroparesis, 240-241
GDM. See *Gestational diabetes mellitus.*
Gemfibrozil (Lopid), 227
Gender, type 2 diabetes and, *12,* 15
Genetics and diabetes, 15-16, 19, 31t
   diagnosis and, 39
   family history in, 76
   hereditary insulin resistance and, 19-20
   in twins, 32
Gestational diabetes mellitus (GDM)
   distinguishing characteristics of, 29, 30t
   fetal risks in, 36
   fructosamine monitoring in, 159
   impaired glucose tolerance risk in, 36
   as indicator for diabetes screening, 39
   prevalence of, 36
   screening for, 36, 42
   type 2 diabetes risk in, 36-37, 77-78
Glargine (Lantus), 138, 141-142
   administration regimens using, 128t
   dosage of, 144
   forgetting to take, 144
   with oral agents, 142
   pharmacokinetics of, 126t, *127,* 142
   side effects of, 144
   structure of, 141
   switching from insulin pump to, 143
   switching from multiple daily injection to, 143
   switching from split-mixed regimen to, 142-143
Glimepiride (Amaryl). See also *Sulfonylureas.*
   availability of, 102
   dosage and pharmacokinetics of, 82t, 104
Glipizide (glucotrol). See also *Sulfonylureas.*
   availability of, 102
   dosage and pharmacokinetics of, 82t, 104
   indications for, 104-105
Glitazones, 78. See also specific drug, eg, *Troglitazone.*
Glucagon, 206
Glucagon-like peptide analogues, 116-117
Glucagonoma, 31t
Glucocorticoids
   diabetes secondary to, 31t
   production of, ketoacidosis and, 190
Glucometer blood glucose monitors, 167t, 171t-172t
Glucophage. See *Metformin.*
Glucose level in blood
   alcohol intake and, 63
   in assessment of therapy effectiveness, 155-157, 156t
   in diabetes warranty program, *44*
   fasting, 35. See also *Impaired fasting glucose.*
      acceptable, with elevated glycohemoglobin, 112
      ADA guidelines for, 73t, 150t
      in diabetes diagnosis, 41t
      in dysmetabolic syndrome, 48t-49t
      in hyperglycemia, 70

14

Glucose level in blood, fasting *(continued)*
    impaired, 24, 35. See also *Impaired glucose tolerance.*
    therapeutic goals for, 156t
  in ketoacidosis, 194t, 198
  measurement of. See *Self-monitoring of blood glucose.*
  normal values in, 40t, 73t, 150t, 156t
  postprandial. See also *Hyperglycemia, postprandial.*
    ADA guidelines for, 73t, 150t
    measurement of, timing of, 72, 157
    normal, 150t
    therapeutic goals for, 72, 156t
  preprandial
    ADA guidelines for, 73t, 150t
    normal, 150t
  therapeutic goals for, 156t
  in type 2 diabetes management, 156-157
  weekly recording of, 178, *180-181*
Glucose production, in liver
  in hyperglycemia pathophysiology, 22, *23,* 70-71
  impaired glucose tolerance and, 19
  reversibility of, 19
Glucose tolerance, impaired. See *Impaired glucose tolerance.*
Glucose tolerance testing, oral, 34t
  fasting plasma glucose testing vs, 23-24
  for impaired glucose tolerance, 23-24
  timing of, 40, 40t
Glucose toxicity, 111. See also *Hyperglycemia.*
  hyperglycemia and, 69
  insulin for, 113
  ketoacidosis and, 190-191
  oral antidiabetic agents for, 114
Glucosidase inhibitors. See *α-glucosidase inhibitors.*
Glucotrol. See *Glipizide.*
GlucoWatch, 185
Glutamic acid decarboxylase, antibodies to, 122, 139
Glyburide (DiaBeta, Glynase PresTab, Micronase). See also *Sulfonylureas.*
  availability of, 102
  contraindications for, 103-104
  dosage and pharmacokinetics of, 82t, 105
  metformin with, 97
Glycated hemoglobin. See *Hemoglobin A_{1C}, glycated.*
Glycated proteins, 159-160
Glycemic control. See *Glucose level in blood.*
Glycet. See *Miglitol.*
Glynase PresTab. See *Glyburide.*
Gum disease, 210

Health Outcomes Prevention Evaluation (HOPE) trial, 217
Heart disease. See also *Cardiovascular disorders; Macrovascular disorders.*
  death from, *17*
Heart failure, congestive, 244
Hemochromatosis, 31t
  erectile dysfunction and, 245
Hemoglobin A_{1C} (HbA_{1C}), glycated
  ADA guidelines for, 73t, 150t
  elevated with acceptable fasting glucose level, oral antidiabetic agents
      for, 112
  false readings of, 158-159
  fructosamine level correlation with, 160, *161*

Hemoglobin A_{1C} *(continued)*
  measurement of, 158-159
  multiple insulin injection regimens for, 137t
  postprandial hyperglycemia and, 71
  process of, 158
  sulfonylurea dosage and, 103
  therapeutic goals for, 150t, 156t
  thiazolidinediones and, 81
Hemolytic anemia, false glycated hemoglobin reading and, 158
Hepatic glucose production. See *Glucose production, in liver.*
Herb supplementation, 59t, 63
HHNS. See *Hyperosmolar hyperglycemic nonketotic syndrome.*
HMG-CoA reductase inhibitors, 227
  for dysmetabolic syndrome, 48
  lipoprotein levels and, 226t
Home monitoring. See also *Self-monitoring of blood glucose.*
  advances in, 179, 185-186
  of glycated proteins, 159-160
  of glycosylated hemoglobin, 159
HOPE (Health Outcomes Prevention Evaluation) trial, 217
Humalog. See *Lispro.*
Huntington's chorea, 31t
Hydronephrosis, 234
Hyperglycemia. See also *Glucose toxicity; Hyperosmolar hyperglycemic nonketotic syndrome.*
  fasting, 70
  insulin resistance and, 20, 69, 80-81
  ketoacidosis and, 34, 190-191
  pathophysiology of, 22, *23,* 70-71
  postprandial, 71-72
    carbohydrate complexity and, 98
  premeal, adjustment of, 177t
  SMBG detection of, 163, 177t, 178
Hyperinsulinemia
  causes of, 20
  circulating, 104
  compensatory, 121
  weight gain from, 145
Hyperkalemia
  ACE inhibitors and, 217
  bicarbonate therapy for, 198
Hyperlipidemia. See *Dyslipidemia; Lipoprotein level.*
Hyperosmolality
  in HHNS, 199
  ketoacidosis and, 191
Hyperosmolar hyperglycemic nonketotic syndrome (HHNS)
  cardiovascular disorders in, 203
  death from, 198
  in elderly people, 198
  laboratory values in, 199, 200t-201t, 202
  pathophysiology of, 199
  symptoms and signs of, 199, 200t-201t, 202
  treatment of, 202-203
  undiagnosed type 2 diabetes and, 198
Hyperprolactinemia, 245
Hypertension
  complications of, 213
  as diabetes type 2 risk factor, 76
  in dysmetabolic syndrome, 48t-49t

14

Hypertension *(continued)*
  exercise in, 213
  as indicator for diabetes screening, 40
  nephropathy and, 234, 236
  treatment of, 214, 217, 237
    blood pressure goal in, 213
    drugs for. See *Antihypertensive agents.*
    weight loss in, 213
  in type 2 diabetes treatment, 156t
Hypertriglyceridemia, 219. See also *Triglyceride level.*
  drugs for, 227
  as indicator for diabetes screening, 40
Hypoaldosteronism, hyporeninemic, 217
Hypoglycemia
  differential diagnosis of, 193
  in elderly people, 163
  etiology of, 203
  during exercise, 66
  from insulin therapy, 145-146
  nocturnal, 205, 207
  prevention of, 206-207
  progression of, 205
  signs of, 204-205
  SMBG detection of, 163, 206
  sulfonylurea-induced, 103
  treatment of, 205-206
Hypotension, orthostatic, 244

IDDM. See *Diabetes mellitus type 1.*
Impaired fasting glucose, 24, 35. See also *Glucose level in blood, fasting.*
Impaired glucose tolerance (IGT)
  diagnostic criteria for, 34t
  distinguishing characteristics of, 31t
  GDM progression to, 36
  hepatic glucose production and, 19
  as indicator for diabetes screening, 40
  macrovascular disease susceptibility in, 35
  prevalence of, 34
  progression to type 2 diabetes, 22, 35
  screening for, 31t23-24
InCharge glucose monitor, 160, 167t, 172t
Incidence of diabetes, 13, *14,* 15-16
Indapamide, 237
Indian(s). See *Asian Indians; Native Americans.*
Indian Health Services (IHS), 257. See also *Native Americans.*
Infections, 39, 207, 208t-209t
  ketoacidosis and, 190
Influenza, death from, *17*
Inhaled insulin therapy, 144-145
Insulin analogs. See specific drug, eg, *Glargine.*
Insulin aspart. See *Aspart.*
Insulin glargine. See *Glargine.*
Insulin lispro. See *Lispro.*
Insulin pump therapy, 128t, 178
  dosage of, 196
  in ketoacidosis, 171
  switching to glargine from, 143
  for type 2 diabetes, 138-139
Insulin receptor abnormalities, diabetes secondary to, 31t

Insulin resistance
  compensated, 20
  in diabetes natural history, 22
  in dysmetabolic syndrome, 49t
  hereditary, 19-20
  hyperglycemia and, 20, 69, 80-81
  in lean vs obese type 2 diabetes, 69-71
  peripheral, in skeletal muscle, 70
  reduction of, 149
  risk factors for, 43, 46
  in tissue, 43
Insulin secretagogues, nonsulfonylurea, 205-106
Insulin secretion
  drug alteration of, 163
  impaired, 19
    hyperglycemia and, 20, 71
    in lean vs obese type 2 diabetes, 700
  ketoacidosis and, 190
  in type 2 diabetes, 32
Insulin sensitizers, 78
Insulin therapy
  aerosolized, 145
  alcohol intake and, 64
  combined with oral agents, 90, *92,* 98, 128t, *153*
    C-peptide values and, 130-131
    dose calculation in, 131-134, 132t-133t
    effectiveness of, 134-135
    injection timing in, 131-132
    for obese vs lean patients, 130-131
    patient selection for, 130-131
    rationale for, 129-130
    SMBG in, 133, 133t
  common regimens for, 128t, 137t
  complications of, 145-146
  continuous subcutaneous. See *Insulin pump therapy.*
  dosage of
    adjustment in, 178-179, 184t
    ketoacidosis and, 191
  exercise during, 66
  for glucose toxicity, 113
  in HHNS, 203
  hypoglycemia from, 145
  inhaled, 144-145
  initiation of, 136, 137t, 138
  insulin preparations for
    basel, 126t
    fixed mixtures, 126t
    human, 124
    interval between injection and effects of, 126t
    mealtime, 126t
    patient variables and, 125
    time course of, 126t
  intensive, 72-74, 76
    adverse effects of, 74, 76
    algorithm form for, *182-183*
    complication reduction and, 72
    DCCT recommendations for, 151, 211-212
    indications for, 127, 129
    injection site for, 129

14

Insulin therapy *(continued)*
   limitations of, 129
      in nutrition therapy, 58t
      in obese patients, 136
      patient education before, 129
      UKPDS recommendations for, 73, 74t, 151, 212
   in ketoacidosis, 196-197
   in multiple injections, 128t, 135-136, 137t, 178
      in obese patients, 136
      in type 1 vs type 2 diabetes patients, 135-136
   oral, 145
   by pump. See *Insulin pump therapy.*
   rationale for, 121-122
   removing patients from, 115-116
   in single injection, 128t, 178
   SMBG during, 133t, 133-134, 163, 177-178
   temporary, 80
      for glucose toxicity, 113
   timing of, 121, 206-207
   in treatment algorithm, *153*
   weight gain from, 145
Intensive therapy
   with insulin. See *Insulin therapy, intensive.*
   non-insulin, 72-73
International Diabetes Center (IDC), 257-258
International Diabetes Federation (IDF), 258
Intracavernosal injections, for erectile dysfunction, 247
Irbesartan, 237
Ischemic heart disease, death from, *17*
Islet cell antibody positivity, 122
Islet cell transplantation, 146-147

Joslin Diabetes Center, 258
Juvenile Diabetes Foundation (JDF) International, 259

Ketoacidosis, 30t
   differential diagnosis of, 192-193
   drug-induced, 163
   in elderly people, 191
   electrolyte depletion in, 190, 196
   etiology of, 189-190
   hyperglycemia and, 34, 190-191
   infections and, 190
   insulin dosage and, 191
   laboratory values in, 194t-195t, 200t-201t
   in malnutrition-related diabetes, 30t, 33-34
   pathophysiology of, 191
   precipitating factors for, 190-191
   subcutaneous insulin pump in, 197
   symptoms and signs of, 191-193, 192t
   treatment of
      bicarbonate in, 198
      fluid and electrolyte replacement in, 196-197
      glucose concentrations and, 196
      goals of, 193
      insulin in, 196-197
      mistakes in, 197
      phosphate replacement in, 197

Ketone bodies
  home measuring of, 160
  in ketoacidosis, 194t
Ketosis, 32, 190
  in HHNS, 199
  treatment of, 198
  in type 1 diabetes, 37
Kidney/pancreas transplantation, 146-147
Kussmaul's respiration, 192, 192t, 199

Lactic acidosis, 96
Lactic dehydrogenase, in ketoacidosis, 195t
Lantus. See *Glargine.*
Late-onset insulin-dependent diabetes mellitus, 113
Latinos, type 2 diabetes in, 11, 15, 77
Lean type 2 diabetes. See *Diabetes mellitus type 2, lean.*
Lente
  administration regimens using, 128t
  dosage of, in combined therapy, 132
  indications for, 124-125
  pharmacokinetics of, 125, 126t, *127*
Lipitor (atorvastatin), 224, 228
Lipodystrophic syndromes, 31t
Lipoprotein level. See also *Dyslipidemia.*
  alcohol intake and, 63
  in diabetes warranty program, *44*
  in dysmetabolic syndrome, 48t
  fat intake and, 59
  fructose intake and, 61
  high-density, 221t
  home measuring of, 160
  ideal, 221t
  intermediate-density, 220
  low-density, 220, 221t
    calculation of, 220
    elevated, drugs for, 227-228
    treatment decisions and, 222t, 225t-226t
  metformin effects on, 95
  protein intake and, 57
  in type 2 diabetes patient
    obesity and, 111
    treatment and, 156t
  very low-density, 219
    gemfibrozil and, 227
Lisinopril, CALM study of, 217
Lispro (Humalog), 122, 124
  administration regimens using, 128t
  advantages of, 124
  benefits of, 141
  indications for, 124-125
  in multiple injection regimens, 138
  neutral protamine lispro (NPL) with, 141
  pharmacokinetics of, *123*, 126t, 140, 142
  premixed formulations of, 140-141
  switching to glargine from, 142-143
Liver
  glucose production in. See *Glucose production, in liver.*
  insulin resistance in, 70
Liver disease, oral antidiabetic agents in, 80

14

Lomotil (diphenoxylate), 243
Loop diuretics. See *Diuretics.*
Lopid (gemfibrozil), 227
Losartan, 237
Lovastatin, 224
Lower extremity
  neuropathy of, 240
  vascular ulcers of, 209t

Macrovascular disorders, 213-228. See also *Cardiovascular disorders;*
    Hypertension; Lipoprotein level.
  death from, 212-213
  in impaired glucose tolerance, 35
  in undiagnosed type 2 diabetes, 13
Macular edema, 229, 233t
Malnutrition, ketoacidosis and, 190
Malnutrition-related diabetes mellitus, 30t, 34
Maturity-onset diabetes of the young (MODY), 37
Mayo Clinic Health Oasis, 259
Mealtime insulins, 126t
Medisense 2 blood glucose monitors, 167t-168t, 172t
Medtronic continuous glucose monitoring system, 186
Meglitinide, 82t, 105-106. See also *Repaglinide (Prandin).*
Metabolic acidosis, 193
Metabolic syndrome. See *Dysmetabolic syndrome.*
Metformin (Glucophage)
  action mechanisms of, 94
  in combination therapy, 86, *87,* 95, 97-99
  contraindications for, 96
  dosage of, 83t, 96-97
  in DPP study, 76
  effectiveness of, *87-88*
  extended release, 97
  glyburide with, 97
  indications for, 79, *152-153*
  in intensive therapy, 93
  lipid effects of, 95
  for obese type 2 diabetes patient, 95
    with/without dyslipidemia, 111
  for patients with acceptable fasting glucose but elevated
    glycohemoglobin, 112
  pharmacokinetics of, 83t
  for prediabetic impaired glucose tolerance, 24
  with/without rosiglitazone, 86, *87*
  side effects of, 96
  in TRIPOD study, 78
Metoclopramide, 242
Metronidazole, 243
Microalbumin in urine
  in diabetes warranty program, *45*
  home measuring of, 160
Micronase. See *Glyburide.*
Microvascular disorders. See also *Nephropathy; Neuropathy; Retinopathy.*
  intensive therapy and, 73-74, 74t
  prevention of, DCCT recommendations for, 211
Miglitol (Glycet), 79. See also *α-glucosidase inhibitors.*
  action mechanisms of, 99, 101
  dosage of, 84t, 101
  patient instructions for, 100t

278

Miglitol (Glycet) *(continued)*
    for patients with acceptable fasting glucose but elevated
        glycohemoglobin, 112
    pharmacokinetics of, 84t, 99, 101
    side effects of, 101
Mineral supplementation, 59t, 62-63
MiniMed GCMS blood glucose monitor, 168t, 172t
Monitoring at home. See *Home monitoring; Self-monitoring of blood glucose.*
Mononeuropathy, 238t, 240
Monounsaturated fat intake, 58t, 60
Mortality in type 2 diabetes, *17*
Muscular dystrophy, 31t
Myocardial infarction
    female protection against, loss of in diabetes, 43
    intensive therapy and, 73, 74t
    type 2 diabetes and
        undiagnosed, 13
        vs nondiabetic, 43

Narcotic analgesics, 239
Nateglinide (Starlix), 83t
    action mechanism of, 106
    dosage of, 108
    effectiveness of, 107-108, *109*
    pharmacokinetics of, 107
    side effects of, 109-110
National Cholesterol Education Program (NCEP), dyslipidemia dietary
        guidelines of, 223
National Diabetes Data Group (NDDG), classification system of, 29, 30t-31t
National Diabetes Education Initiative (NDEI), 259-260
National Diabetes Education Program (NDEP), 260
National Eye Institute (NEI), 260
National Health Council, 260
National Institute of Diabetes and Digestive and Kidney Diseases
        (NIDDK), 261
National Kidney Foundation, 261
National Stroke Association (NSA), 262
Native Americans. See *American Indians.*
    resources for, 257
    type 2 diabetes in, 77
        diagnosis of, 39
        prevalence of, 11, 15, 32
Natural history of type 2 diabetes, 22-25, *23*
    insulin resistance in, 81
    insulin therapy and, 122
    intensive therapy and, 74, *75*
Nephropathy
    ACE inhibitors and, 216t
    detection of, 233-236
    in diabetes warranty program, *45*
    hyperglycemia and, 234
    hypertension and, 213, 236
    incidence of, 233
    pathophysiology of, 233-234
    patient education on, 235-236
    potassium restriction in, 63
    protein intake and, 57

14

Nephropathy *(continued)*
  treatment of
    glycemic control in, 236-237
    hypertension management in, 237
    protein intake restriction in, 238
Nerve stimulation, transcutaneous (TENS), 240
Neurogenic bladder, 243
  nephropathy and, 234
Neurontin (gabapentin), 239
Neuropathy
  amyotrophy as, 240
  autonomic, 238t
  drugs for, 239-240
  gastropariesis as, 240, 242-243
  in HHNS, 202
  incidence of, 238
  management algorithm for, *241*
  mononeuropathy as, 238t, 240
  sensorimotor peripheral, 238t
  symmetric distal, 238t, 239-240
  transcutaneous nerve stimulation for, 240
Neutral protamine Hagedorn (NPH)
  administration regimens using, 128t
  advantages of, 124
  dosage of, in combined therapy, 132
  indications for, 124-125
  pharmacokinetics of, 126t, *127*
  switching to glargine from, 142-143
Niaspan, 227
Nicotinic acid, 227
  diabetes secondary to, 34t
  lipoprotein levels and, 226t, 228
NIDDM. See *Diabetes mellitus type 2.*
Nocturia, 210
Nocturnal hypoglycemia, 205, 207
Nonsteroidal anti-inflammatory drugs. See also *Aspirin.*
  nephropathy and, 234, 239
Norepinephrine production, 190
Novolog. See *Aspart.*
NPH. See *Neutral protamine Hagedorn.*
Nutrition therapy
  alcohol intake in, 58t, 63
  behavior modification in, 54
  body weight considerations in, 53-54
  calorie intake in, 55t, 56
  carbohydrate intake in, 58t, 60-61
  in diabetes warranty program, *45*
  dietary changes in, 53
  dietary habit and intake assessment in, 51-52
  dietitian consult in, 52-53
  for dyslipidemia, 222t, 223, 224t-225t
  fasting blood glucose level and, 52
  fat intake in, 58t, 59-60
  fat substitutes in, 62
  fructose intake in, 61
  goals of, 51
  insulin with, 58t
  nutritive/nonnutritive sweeteners in, 62
  oral antidiabetic agents with, 79

Pregnancy
    diabetes onset in. See *Gestational diabetes mellitus.*
    diabetes risk assessment in, 42
    eye care before and during, 232
    oral antidiabetic agents in, 80, *152*
    postprandial hyperglycemia in, 71
Prestige glucose monitors, 168t, 173t
Prevalence of type 2 diabetes, 11, 32
    age and, 11, *12*
    gender and, *12*
    race/ethnicity and, 11-12
Priapism, 247
Primary care provider, in diabetes prevention, 24-25
Propoxyphene, 239
Prostaglandins, 247
Protein(s)
    glycated, 159-160
    in urine, in diabetes warranty program, *45*
Protein intake
    nephropathy and, 57, 238
    recommended daily allowance of, 57
Psychological issues, in erectile dysfunction, 244
Psychosocial support, in nutrition therapy, 54
Pulmonary safety studies, in inhaled insulin therapy, 144-145

Quality of life in type 2 diabetes, 210
    neuropathy and, 238-240
Questran, 224

Race/ethnicity and type 2 diabetes, 77. See also specific ethnic group.
    in diagnosis, 39
    etiologic sequence in, 21
    GDM and, 36, 42
    impaired glucose tolerance progression to, 34-35
    insulin therapy and, 122
    prevalence of, 11-12, 15, 32
Radiocontrast dyes, nephropathy and, 234
Ramipril, 217
ReliOn blood glucose monitor, 169t, 174t
Renal disorders. See *Nephropathy.*
Renal tubular acidosis, 217
Repaglinide (Prandin), 79. See also *Meglitinide.*
    action mechanisms of, 105
    in combination therapy, 106
    dosage and pharmacokinetics of, 82t, 106
    exercise and, 66
    for lean type 2 diabetes, 113
    for patients with acceptable fasting glucose but elevated
        glycohemoglobin, 112
    side effects of, 106
    for thin elderly patients, 112
Resources for diabetes, 258-262
Retinopathy. See also *Visual blurring.*
    blindness from, 229
    early detection of, 228
    evaluation and referral in, 231-232, 233t
    hypertension and, 213
    nonproliferative, 229, *230*
    patient education on, 229

14

Retinopathy *(continued)*
    preproliferative, 230, *231*
    proliferative, 230-231
    treatment of, 232-233
Rezulin (troglitazone), 77, 81, 85
Risk factors for type 2 diabetes, 20, 24, 39-40. See also specific risk
        factor, eg, *Obesity.*
Rosiglitazone (Avandia), 79. See also *Thiazolidinediones.*
    anti-inflammatory effects of, 89
    blood pressure and, 89
    in combination therapy, 85-90
    in diabetes type 2 prevention, 78
    dosage of, 83t, 85-91, 86
    effect on C-peptide, insulin, and proinsulin levels, 85
    effectiveness of, 85-98, *87-88*
    insulin-sparing pancreatic effect of, 86
    insulin with, 90
    lipoprotein levels and, 89
    metformin with/without, 86, *87-88*
    pharmacokinetics of, 83t, 85
    side effects of, 90-91
    sulfonylurea with, 86
    urinary albumin excretion and, 89

Saccharin, 62
Salt restriction, 59t, 213
Scandinavian Simvastatin Survival Study (4S), 226t
Screening for type 2 diabetes, indications for, 39-40
Scrotal infection, 208t
Secondary diabetes mellitus, 30t-31t, 33
Sedentary lifestyle. See also *Exercise.*
    calorie intake calculation in, 56
    type 2 diabetes and
        etiologic sequence in, 20
        impaired glucose tolerance progression to, 35
Self-monitoring of blood glucose (SMBG), 156-157. See also
        Home monitoring.
    accuracy of, 160-161, 165
    advances in, 179, 185-186
    advantages and disadvantages of, 157, 164-165
    DCCT and UKPDS recommendations for, 162
    equipment for, 166t-174t, 179, 185-186
    before and after exercise, 66
    frequency of, 162, 165, 175-178
    for glycated hemoglobin, 158-159
    for glycated proteins, 159-160
    hyperglycemia detection by, 163, 177t, 178
    hypoglycemia detection by, 163, 206
    implantable sensors for, 186
    indications for, 175
    infrared technology in, 186
    in initiation of insulin therapy, 136, 138
    insulin dosage adjustment and, 178-179, 184t
    in insulin therapy combined with oral agents, 131-133
    log book in, 178, *180-181*
    for nutrition therapy planning, 454
    as part of regimen, 163
    patient education in, 162, 229, 265
    by patients who do not take insulin, 176

Self-monitoring of blood glucose (SMBG) *(continued)*
    by patients who take insulin, 177t, 177-178
    procedures in, 160
    rationale for, 162-163
    sucrose intake and, 61
    sulfonylurea dosage and, 104
    therapeutic effectiveness and, 155, 156t
    timing of, 40, 40t, 157
Semmes Weinstein monofilaments, 248
Sickle cell trait, false glycated hemoglobin reading and, 158
Sildenafil (Viagra), 247
    action mechanism of, 245
    contraindications for, 246
    dosage of, 245-246
    effectiveness of, 246
    side effects of, 246
Simvastatin, 224
Skeletal muscle, peripheral insulin resistance in, 70
Sof-Tact blood glucose monitor, 169t, 174t
Starlix (nateglinide), 83t
Stop Non–Insulin-dependent Diabetes Mellitus Study, 78
Stress, ketoacidosis and, 190
Stroke
    differential diagnosis of, 192-193
    undiagnosed type 2 diabetes and, 13
Sucrose intake
    in nutrition therapy, 58t
    SMBG and, 61
Sugar alcohol intake, 62
Sulfonylureas. See also specific drugs.
    action mechanisms of, 101
    alcohol intake and, 64
    availability of, 101-102
    characteristics of, 82t
    in combination therapy, 94-94, *153*
    contraindications for, 103-104, 111
    dosage of, 103
    effectiveness of, 101-102
    exercise and, 66
    for glucose toxicity, 103, 114
    insulin with temporarily, 103
    in intensive therapy, 73
    for lean patients, elderly, 112
    lean patients, with type 2 diabetes, 113
    as monotherapy, *152*
    in obese patient with/without dyslipidemia, 111
    rosiglitazone with, 86
    side effects of, 102-104
Supreme II blood glucose monitor, 169t, 174t
Sweeteners, nutritive/nonnutritive, 62
Symmetric distal neuropathy, 238t, 239

Tachycardia, 244
Taking Control of Your Diabetes, 262
Testosterone therapy, 245
Thiazide diuretics
    in combination therapy, 219
    insulin secretion and, 163

14

Thiazide diuretics *(continued)*
  potential benefits of, 216t, 218
  side effects of, 188t, 245
Thiazolidinediones
  action mechanisms of, 80
  characteristics of, 83t
  in combination therapy, 81, 106
  indications for, 79, *152-153*
  for obese type 2 diabetes patient with/without dyslipidemia, 111
  for patients with acceptable fasting glucose but elevated
      glycohemoglobin, 112
  PPAR activation by, 81
  for prediabetic impaired glucose tolerance, 24
  for thin elderly patients, 112
Thin persons with type 2 diabetes. See *Diabetes mellitus type 2, lean.*
Thrifty Gene Hypothesis, 16
Thyroid function tests, in diabetes warranty program, *45*
Tolazamide (Tolinase), 82t, 101. See also *Sulfonylureas.*
Tolbutamide (Orinase), 82t, 101
Tramadol (Ultram), 239-240
Transcutaneous nerve stimulation (TENS), 240
Transplantation
  of islet cells, 146-147
  of kidney, 146-147
  of pancreas, 147
Treat to Target study, 142
Treatment of type 2 diabetes. See also specific treatment, eg, *Antidiabetic*
      agents, oral.
  algorithm for, *152-153*
  assessment of
    glycated hemoglobin in, 159
    other glycated proteins in, 159-160
    plasma glucose concentration in. See *Self-monitoring of blood glucose.*
  goals of, 149, 155
  individualized approach to, 149, 151
  methods of, 149
Tricor (fenofibrate), 227
Tricyclic antidepressants, 239
Triglyceride level, 48t, 221t. See also *Hypertriglyceridemia.*
  dietary guidelines and, 223
TRIPOD (Troglitazone in Prevention of Diabetes) study, 78
Troglitazone (Rezulin), 81, 85
  in DPP study, 77
  liver toxicity of, 77, 81, 85
  in TRIPOD study, 78
Troglitazone in Prevention of Diabetes (TRIPOD) study, 78
Twins, diabetes in, 32
Tylenol, for neuropathy, 240

UKPDS. See *United Kingdom Prospective Diabetes Study (UKPDS)*
      recommendations.
Ultralente
  indications for, 124-125
  pharmacokinetics of, 125, 126t, *127*
  regimens using, 128t, 138
  switching to glargine from, 143
Ultram (tramadol), 239
Undiagnosed diabetes, 33
  angina and, 13

286

Undiagnosed diabetes *(continued)*
    diabetic complications and, 13
    HHNS and, 198
    macrovascular disorders and, 13
    prevalence of, 12
United Kingdom Prospective Diabetes Study (UKPDS)
    β-blockers on, 217-218
    combination therapy in, *75*
    intensive insulin therapy in, 73, 151, 212
    microvascular and cardiovascular complications in, oral agents and, 214
    microvascular complications in, 74t
    myocardial infarctions in, 74t
    nephropathy management in, 236
    retinopathy prevalence in, 13
    SMBG in, 162
    structure of, 73, *75*
Uremia, 234-235
    false glycated hemoglobin reading and, 158
Urinary tract infection, 207, 209t, 243
Urine protein/microalbumin, in diabetes warranty program, *45*

Vacuum constrictor devices, for erectile dysfunction, 246-247
Valsartan, 237
Vascular endothelial dysfunction, in dysmetabolic syndrome, 49t
Vascular inflammation, glitazones and, 81
Vascular ulcers, of lower extremity, 209t
Vasodilators, for erectile dysfunction, 247
Vegetable intake, 60, 238
Viagra. See *Sildenafil.*
Visual blurring, 39, 210, 233t. See also *Retinopathy.*
Vitamin supplementation, 59t, 62-63
Vulvovaginitis, 208t

Weight gain. See also *Body fat distribution; Body weight; Obesity.*
    in hyperinsulinemia, 145
    in insulin therapy, 76, 145
    sulfonylurea-induced, 102, 104
Weight loss, 33, 39
    calorie intake formula for, 56
    dietitian consult during, 52-53
    for dysmetabolic syndrome, 47
    emphasis in, 54
    fat intake and, 60
    in hypertension treatment, 213
    oral antidiabetic agents in, 80
    techniques in, 54
    therapeutic effects of, 53
White blood cell count, in ketoacidosis, 195t
World Health Organization (WHO) criteria
    for diabetes, based on oral glucose tolerance testing, 34t, 42
    for impaired glucose tolerance, 34t
Wound healing, 39

Yohimbine, 245

14